PRETTY HAPPY

PRETTY HAPPY

HEALTHY WAYS TO LOVE YOUR BODY

KATE HUDSON

with

BILLIE FITZPATRICK

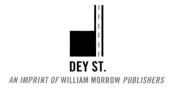

DEY ST.

AN IMPRINT OF WILLIAM MORROW *PUBLISHERS*

The advice herein is not intended to replace the services of
trained health professionals, or be a substitute for medical advice.
You are advised to consult with your heath care professional
with regard to matters relating to your health, and in particular
regarding matters that may require diagnosis or medical attention.

HarperCollins books may be purchased for educational, business,
or sales promotional use. For information please e-mail the
Special Markets Department at SPsales@harpercollins.com.

FIRST EDITION

Designed by Headcase Design
Photographs by Darren Ankenman
Illustrations by Sun Young Park

Library of Congress Cataloging-in-Publication Data
has been applied for.

ISBN 978-0-06-243423-4 (hardcover)
978-0-06-248202-0 (Target edition)
978-0-06-249712-3 (Indigo signed edition)
978-0-06-249707-9 (BAM signed edition)
978-0-06-249708-6 (B&N signed edition)

16 17 18 19 20   OV/QUAD   10 9 8 7 6 5 4 3 2 1

3201 8545

For my children,
who keep me active, vital,
and make me want to live
as long as possible

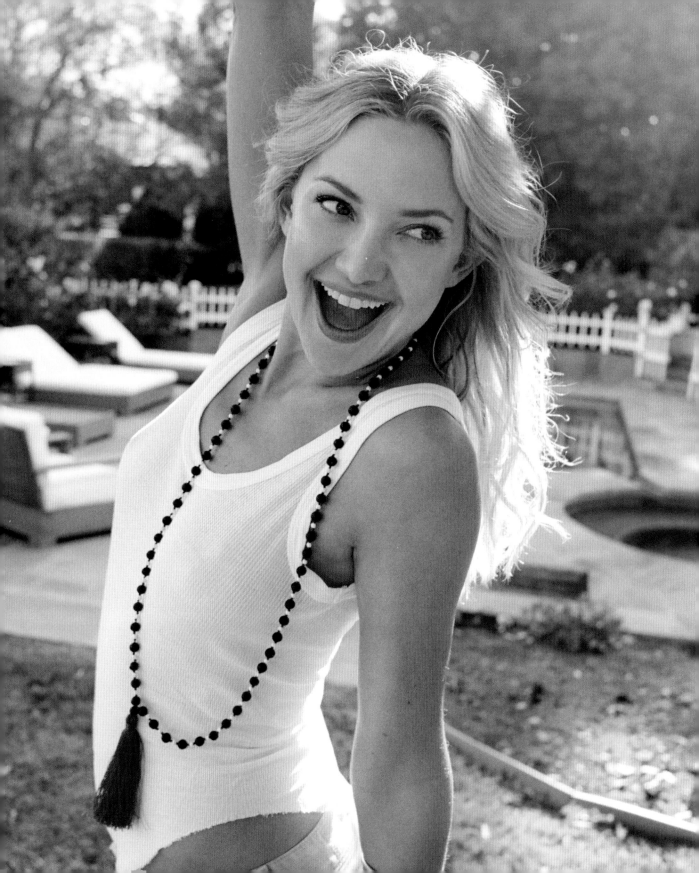

CONTENTS

PART THREE

Living Body Smart

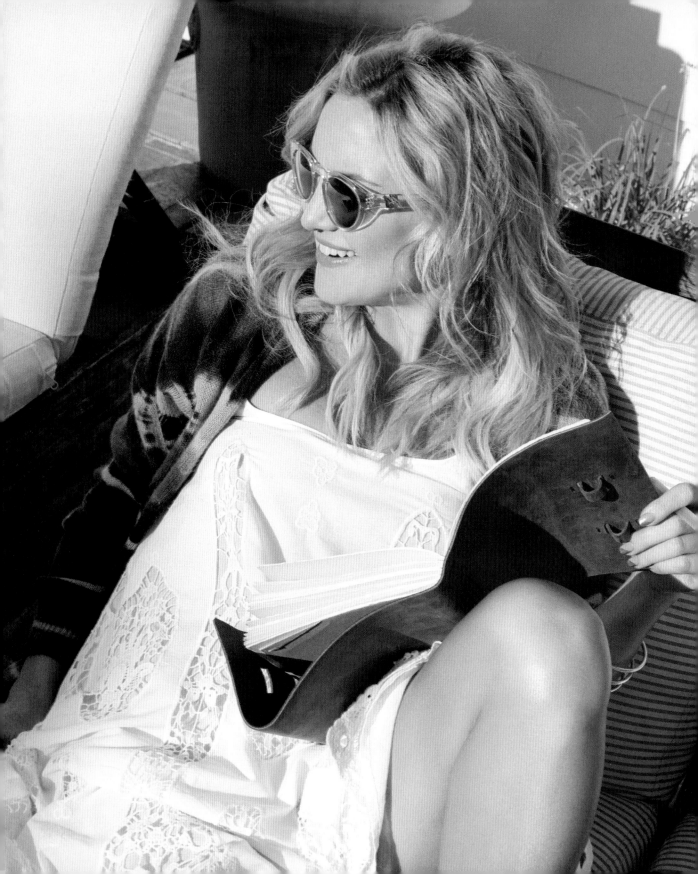

INTRODUCTION

I HOPE THIS ISN'T disappointing, but this book is not meant to be some kind of weird tell-all. Rather, it's a tell-true, focused on how I figured out how to connect to myself, understand what my body needs, and put that information together so I no longer have to worry about or overthink how I eat or how I work out and for how long. I finally feel confident that I have something to share. I want to give others a way to feel as positive and motivated as I try to be, because seeing that I can help makes me feel my best. This book is also about how I learned to slow down and fine-tune how I eat and exercise and practice meditation in a way that grounds me when life gets bumpy.

Why do I feel more confident about what I've learned? Lately, I've been realizing that just as my public roles have changed and evolved, so too have my inner roles—especially my relationship with myself. People may see me as buoyant and always smiling, but the truth is, I'm not always like that. No one is. Like everyone else, I have my good days, my not-so-good days, and my totally awful days. I'm in my midthirties now, and my life is even more complicated and busy, with more and more responsibilities. But I also happen to be more carefree than I was even in my early twenties, before I became a mom. I also feel stronger than ever, more self-assured and more resilient. Does this sound like a contradiction? Let me explain. I guess you can say that I finally feel at peace with myself, ready and willing to take on new challenges, looking forward to the years ahead with fearlessness, confidence, creativity, and lots of humor, not shy or afraid of any upsets that are bound to happen in my lifetime. And I just feel more confident that now I can share some insight, and even if it resonates with only one person, I will have contributed in a positive way.

Another reason I decided to write this book was out of frustration. I'm often asked how I stay in shape. How I lost all that baby weight after my first son, Ryder, was born. How I seem to effortlessly lose ten pounds in preparation for a new film role. How I look and seem so healthy. The responses captured and then reported by the media are typically just sound bites—"I love to jump rope." "I'm into yoga." "I do Pilates." "I'm vegan." "I work out twenty minutes a day." "I work out two and a half hours a day."

It's not that these sound bites aren't true—some are, some are not—but they just don't tell the whole story. And though I understand that nowadays we have become accustomed to getting our information immediately, in bite-size snippets or tweets, learning how to really take care of yourself doesn't happen immediately at all. In other words, if you want to make lifestyle changes, it doesn't happen with a Like on Instagram! It takes time and discipline.

My frustration comes from the fact that learning to take care of yourself will never be captured in a sound bite, just as how I live my life could never be captured in a four-minute interview. So since I really want to spread the word about some of the lessons I've learned and the things I've found that make me feel great, and I can't sit down for a long conversation with you over hot tea, I decided to put my ideas about how to be body smart in this book.

One of the main ideas I came to is that being body smart is an ongoing process, not a diet or a program that begins one day and ends twenty-one days later. Just like yours are, my body and mind are always changing, which means that taking care of myself requires that I tune in regularly, ready to make small adjustments to fit the changes. This idea of constant change was a huge revelation for me! I used to think I could just figure out the best diet for me, that I'd lose weight, stick to that weight, and never have to worry again. But life doesn't work that way—nor does true self-care. I want this book to be a map for you to figure out how to take good care of yourself—mind and body.

I didn't just wake up one day understanding how to take care of myself. I had to learn how to do so over time, and I continue to learn—each and every day. Again, this is a process because my body is constantly changing—so is yours. And when I learned how to accept that it will always be like this, I relaxed. Our bodies do not stand still for time.

Another important lesson I learned, and one that I want you to learn, is that perfection is for amateurs. No, seriously. When you understand yourself and connect to how you can become body smart, you realize pretty quickly that the perfect, the ideal, is not the goal. Instead, the goal is feeling good in your body. That's what leads to confidence, to feeling and looking fit, and being *pretty happy*. Doesn't that sound great? I think so!

You may assume from all the photos and video clips out there that I was born thin, with a sleek, toned body. Ahh—not the case. Like every woman, I work at it and continue to work at it. I've lost weight, gained it right back, and lost it again. I've been thin but not toned, skinny but not strong, and none of the above.

Another realization I've had since Bing, my second son, was born and I launched Fabletics, my workout clothing line, is that I have to take care of myself in a more complete way. I'd use the word *holistic* if it hadn't already been beaten to death. I'd use the word *balanced* if that word, too, hadn't almost lost its meaning. The word that seems most relatable, real, and true is *connected*. I finally feel truly connected within myself—my mind and body, with a little soul thrown in for good measure. Being connected and aware has kept me grounded in my life even though I am always on the move. I feel focused and clearheaded despite continuing to enjoy jumping from one project to the next, one self-help book to another and then back to poetry. I am busy, but I don't feel frenetic. I feel energized yet peaceful. And on the physical side, to find myself in this place after years feels like a triumph. It wasn't until I connected the dots—how I eat, what makes me happy when I exercise, and what I truly need—that my life and my body calmed down.

So it's this place of connection that has inspired me to write this book.

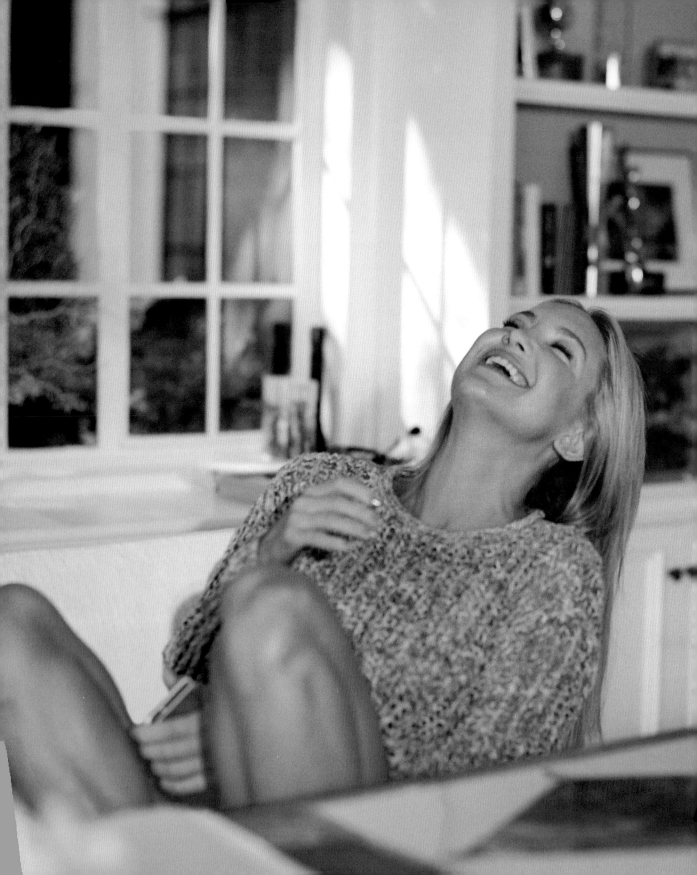

People keep asking me if I have a secret—a secret diet, a secret formula for losing weight, a secret exercise routine that makes me toned, strong, and feeling sexy. Photographs of me or any other celebrity may inspire you, but they won't get you off the couch. That's up to you. Instead, what I want for you is what I discovered for myself: that taking care of yourself is the single most important connection you can make in your life. When you feel calm and in sync with yourself, when you feel sated and neither hungry nor full, when you feel energized by whatever form of exercise puts a smile on your face—that's when you know you've hit the jackpot.

I came to this understanding through trial and error, by constantly changing things up, observing what works for people close to me, including my parents, and doing my own research. Ever since I decided to launch Fabletics and really spread the word about our mission "to live fit and achieve your passions in life," I have been diving into positive psychology, exercise physiology, cutting-edge nutritional science, and brain research that shows how certain foods affect our bodies by setting off dangerous, unhealthy habits, and how physical activity interacts with the brain. My mom, Goldie Hawn, has been working closely with neuroscientists and positive psychologists for some time in her work with MindUP, an important curriculum to help kids de-stress and manage their emotions so they can learn more effectively in school. My mom's work deepened my own curiosity about mindfulness—as a mom myself and as a woman. I did a lot of research, including learning about the benefits of an alkaline diet (as opposed to a diet that is highly acidic), and reached out to a number of mind-body practitioners and experts in the areas of Ayurvedic medicine (an ancient Indian approach to the integration of holistic mind and body health) so that I could create a simple, easy-to-use primer on weight loss, mind-body connection, and fitness to use in my own life. Now you can tailor it for your life, using *Pretty Happy*.

As women, we know it's the details that make the difference. We don't

———

want basic information that seems geared toward the masses, but rather much more personalized, nuanced instruction that helps us understand something new from the inside. We want to internalize what we learn so that it makes sense to us on a personal level. That's how this book will work. First, I'm going to share my *Drawing Board* so you can create your own.

Think of the Drawing Board conceptually—a place to write down all your thoughts, feelings, questions, and fears about your body, but also about your life. That's what I do. It's a kind of living document that keeps me in touch with me. Sometimes my Drawing Board is my journal. Sometimes I do a huge collage board. But really you can use anything you like—a legal pad, a diary, the Notes application in your smartphone. If I feel anxious or stuck, I return to my Drawing Board. If I am elated and joyful, I record it on my Drawing Board. After a run, a meditation, or a particularly difficult day, I go to my Drawing Board and put down my thoughts, my feelings, and the patterns that I see emerging. My Drawing Board is an ever-changing, real-time document of me and where I am in my life so that I always stay connected with myself and those I love. My Drawing Board helps me trust myself.

I will show you how you can create your own Drawing Board and use it to create an intuitive relationship with yourself, one that I think will lead to your own inner balance, sense of connectedness, and inner groundedness. There is no one way to find yourself, but I hope you will discover yours.

Of course, I will share how I eat and stay active, but that is not so you can follow suit exactly. This book is meant to help you find the things you like and decide what works for you. Perhaps you will be inspired; perhaps what you enjoy and what you need will become clearer. I am going to give you reliable information that you can use to make good decisions—ones that work for you.

And although I'll give you some reliable, science-backed strategies for reducing body fat and losing pounds, I'm not giving you a program that makes you look like me.

I promise I am not going to overwhelm you with biology and chemistry. I

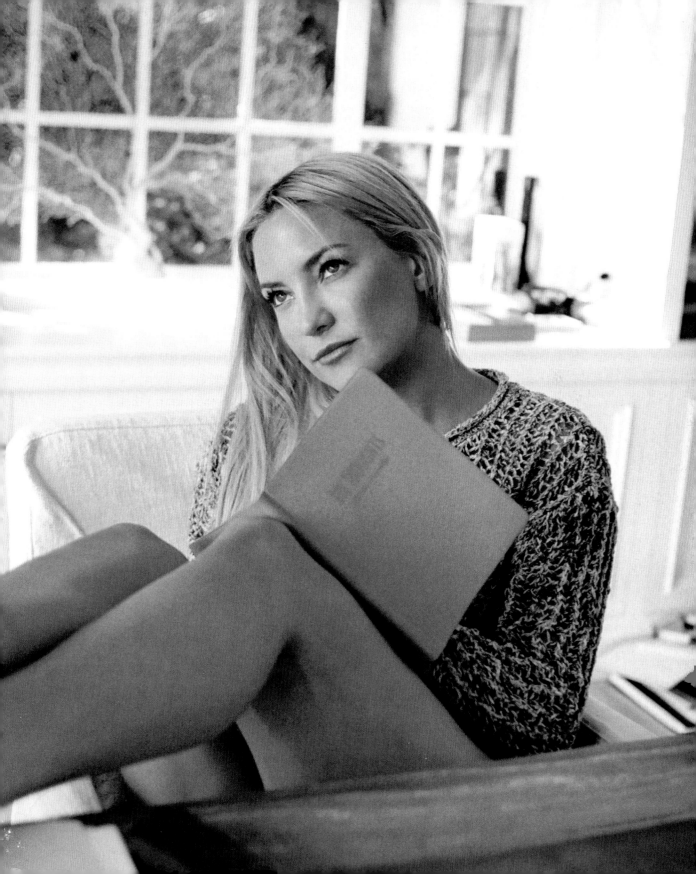

am not going to give you tons of nutritional advice that will make you want to scream. I just want you to know that I've done my homework, culled the most important and valuable takeaways from all my research, and presented it here as easy-to-follow tips, tools, and strategies.

Like anything, learning something truly meaningful takes time and effort. I try to remind myself of that every day I wake up and don't want to work out, don't want to move, don't want to eat clean and well. And I think this is a feeling many of you might relate to—knowing that being happy and finding pleasure and contentment takes discipline.

Just as building Fabletics is the symbol of my internal dialogue about not just reaching for surface results but showing myself that I can dig deeper, I want this book to offer you some ideas for how you can go to that deeper, more real place with yourself. I hope you can find the kind of strength and resilience that I've found in the face of a busy, full life. I hope you can find a sense of connectedness outside yourself, knowing that the more peaceful you are within, the more peaceful you will be in your relationships with others. I'm hoping that you find something inside of yourself—in this book—even if it's one thing to aspire to, one goal in your everyday life. And know that I am deeply respectful of you and wherever you are in your life right now. Believe me, I know making lifestyle changes isn't easy, but we've all got to start some-where. So let's make a pact that we will try to enjoy the process!

So, this book is an invitation from me to you. Why settle for mediocre and frenetic when you can feel simply awesome?! Don't you want to feel grounded in your life and in your body? To feel happy to wake up in the morning and tackle your to-do list or look forward to a day of enjoyment? Don't you want to feel so good in your body that you can skip the mirror and the scale once in a while? That on the days you don't feel great or don't have the tools, you can trust that you can go to your Drawing Board and get back to that right place for you? That's what being body smart is all about.

When you connect with your breath, and nurture a positive, intuitive relationship with yourself and your body, you will begin to settle and feel in sync with everything around you. This is the essence of health. When we can stay well—adapt to greater stress and have greater endurance—then the joy and inspiration rush in, impelling us forward into life.

Taken all together, this hard-earned wisdom is about finding a path to *pretty happy* and joy—which is not a concept but an experience, an attitude, and a goal for every day of your life. Don't wait for happy to happen. Seize the day! Start now! And don't overthink it!

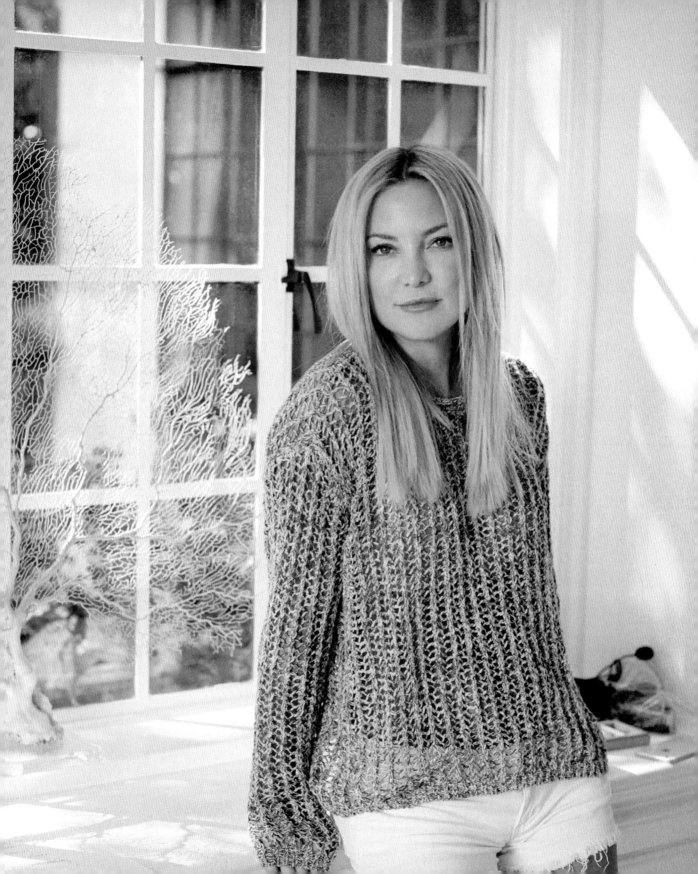

PART ONE

BECOMING BODY SMART

Being body smart means connecting to and honoring your body— where you are now and where you want to be in the future. It means being truly honest with yourself and acknowledging both your strengths and those parts of yourself that can get you into trouble. When you start from this place of acceptance, you set yourself up for true success.

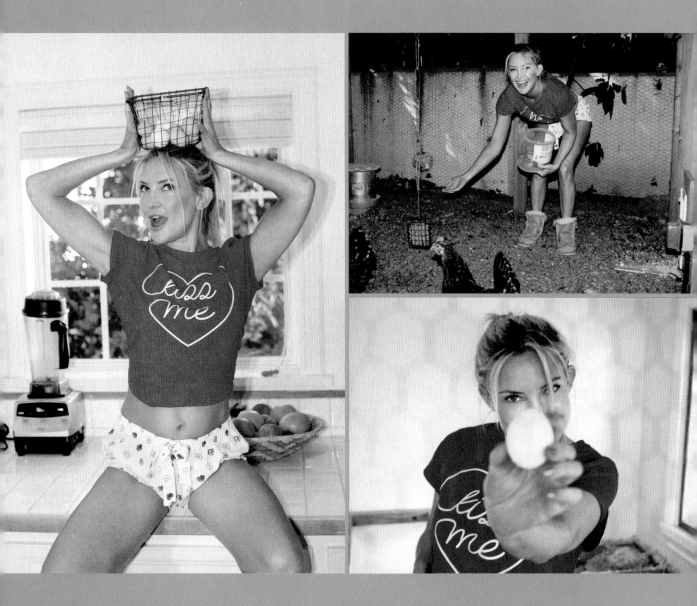

CHAPTER ONE

DON'T CAGE ME IN

What, Me Listen?

I DON'T ALWAYS WORK out, I don't always eat perfectly, and I don't always get enough rest, but I have learned to tune in to how I am feeling—how my clothes feel, how my head feels, what my thoughts and feelings are telling me—and trust these clues to tell me what I need. This tuning in has become an absolute necessity to my overall well-being.

In the past, I went through periods when I felt all I did was muddle through. At hyperspeed, I went from job to job, activity to activity, house to house. I could not settle down. Constant movement was the only thing that made sense to me. The turning point came the first time I hit a wall and felt like I couldn't handle my life. Granted, I was young, still a teenager at nineteen, but my career had started to take off. I had started to get roles in films and begun traveling around the world—Ireland, Toronto, New York City. I was literally away from home for about eighteen months straight. I had not yet accumulated enough income to have my own place, so I lived out of hotels and with friends. When I had a few days back home in Los Angeles, I stayed with my parents.

I was having all these amazing experiences and meeting all sorts of interesting people, but part of me was becoming unhinged. One day I was on a Jetway, ready to take off on yet another flight to god knows where, and I just kind of lost it. As soon as I got to my seat, I called my mom, very upset.

I was homesick. I missed my parents. My family.

All of a sudden the whirlwind had settled and I was feeling insecure, lonely, and young—like I was in over my head and my feet were not at all on the ground.

As only mothers can do, my mom told me to take a deep breath and then squint my eyes.

"I want you to squint your eyes—I want you to squint your eyes really small and get your vision really fuzzy."

"Mom," I moaned. "How is that going to help?"

"Just do it," she said. "Squint your eyes and imagine you're seeing everything around you for the first time."

So I squinted my eyes tightly and began to look around me. Everything looked really small and strange. I found myself staring at a groove on the seat, a hole in the leather on the back of the chair. I looked at the signs around the plane.

And then I started to calm down. I got what my mom was trying to help me understand: Sometimes we just need to slow things down so we can reframe—our situation, our thoughts and feelings, even our lives. And not to take everything so seriously. What she was telling me, and what she explained later on, was not to forget that you are good and that everything is all right. You've been working without a pause and your brain is on overdrive. The *situation* is what feels out of control. You are okay.

That was a huge lesson, one that really was the beginning of me taking responsibility for my own state of mind. I feel lucky to have a mom like that!

So now this process of tuning in, framing or reframing what is going on with me and around me, gives me the feedback I need to take care of myself.

Sometimes the information signals that I'm out of balance somehow. Maybe I spent the day before eating junk food on set, or I've been traveling so much that I haven't exercised in a week. Sometimes I tune in and I realize I'm hungry because I haven't eaten enough. Sometimes the signals indicate that I'm anxious or worried. Sometimes I just need to take a long nap.

My point is this: I trust my body to talk to me. To tell me what it needs and what it doesn't. I trust it to send me signals about whether I am eating well or not so great, whether I'm getting just enough rest and fun. If my body feels tight and achy, I need to carve out more downtime, relax, or try a different type of physical activity. (But if you have a persistent issue, you should seek professional advice or see a specialist.) Sometimes my body tells me very simple things, like that I need to drink more water. Really. These are simple fixes, but they make a huge difference in how I feel on the inside and look on the outside. When I tune in to these sensations and read the emotional and physical signals my body is giving me, I can then begin to process what it is I need, if anything, or what I need to stop if my body is telling me that something is not right. If I have a breakout on my skin, I know it's probably from eating too much refined sugar or a change in hormones. If I feel bloated and irritable, it might mean one of two things: I ate too much sodium or starchy carbs, or my gut is out of whack. (Be forewarned: I'm going to share lots about healthy flora!)

Like a lighthouse at the edge of the ocean, your body signals information about how it is feeling and provides direction for where to go. When we learn to pay attention to the signals our bodies are giving us, we have a better chance of making healthier, cleaner choices about what we eat and what we do, and resisting the foods and activities that deplete us.

I also pay attention to the signals of my heart and mind. Am I so stressed that I can't even focus on work or be patient with my kids? Am I so reactive that I seem to jump out of my skin when someone speaks to me?

Listening to my body and mind, learning to understand the cues and signals, has become the single most important way for me to take care of myself.

It's how I lose weight when I need to. It's how I keep myself toned and strong. It's also how I stay grounded and connected—in my head, heart, and soul.

But let me be clear: I don't treat my body as some kind of delicate temple—no—I'm way too busy, way too practical for that. I'm also not trying to be perfect, because perfection is too subjective to measure.

What I've done is create a relationship with my body that is based on the idea that all of us—our bodies—possess natural intelligence. Bodies and brains are designed to eat and digest a wide array of foods so that we get enough basic nutrients to function optimally. Without these basics, the body's systems will malfunction—the body will gain weight, it will bloat, it will become irregular and slow, it will develop inflammation and pain, it will not sleep. These signs of illness or distress are the body's way of telling us something's wrong—with what we are eating, how much or little we are eating, whether we are eating foods that our bodies can neither process nor absorb. Our bodies will eventually break down when they are not given what they need (i.e., nutrition) or when they are inundated with toxins that interfere with proper functioning.

Since we are each distinct individuals, our food and nutrient needs vary, as do our bodies' abilities to withstand toxins, stimuli, and bad food choices. So yes, we all need the basic vitamins, minerals, protein, fats, carbohydrates, and water to survive. But there is no one precise way to obtain these nutrients. Of course this makes sense—think of all the world's amazing cultures and how varied their cuisines are!

This is why I would never declare one way to eat is the best way—I won't assume that you share my taste buds!

The same is true of exercise. What I do for fun reflects what gives me pleasure. And, as you may have gathered from photos, I like all kinds of things. My choices are constantly changing! An adventurer at heart, I probably will try anything once—from surfing to mountain climbing. But what I enjoy doing matters less than what *you* enjoy doing.

If you want to really own your body and honor it, you need to spend time playing around and finding what *you* enjoy. You don't have to already be good at something—feel free to be a beginner and try a new activity! But the truth of the matter is this: If you want to feel in sync with your body, you need to get it moving. Our bodies are designed to move, and without daily activity, they will begin to break down.

It's Never One Size Fits All

WE ALL KNOW—FROM years of personal experience and the existence of thousands of diet programs, fitness crazes, books, and gurus—that there is no one diet or exercise plan that works for all people. Atkins, Mediterranean, Paleo, The Whole30, vegan, raw, CrossFit, TRX, Barre, Pilates—you name it. Any diet will work if all you want is to lose weight. Any fitness plan will work, at first, if you stick to it for a while. But if you want to create an intimate relationship with your body, understand its needs and wants, what it likes (what makes you feel energized and satisfied) and what it doesn't like (what it reacts negatively to), then I'd like to share some tips with you. Read on if:

* You want to find that inner trust that centers and guides you.

* You want to tune in to yourself so you don't have to overthink what you eat every day.

* You want to integrate movement into your daily life in a way that makes you feel vital, strong, and in control.

* You want to find peace of mind and calm so you can sleep well and wake rested.

* You want to be able to listen to your body when it speaks to you.

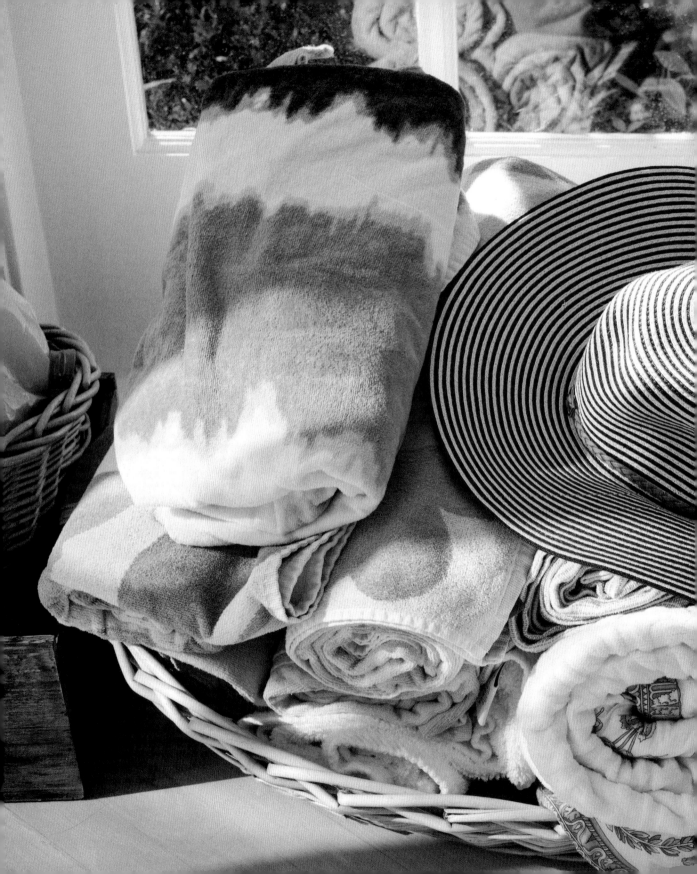

Life is a verb.
—Charlotte Perkins Gilman

It Takes a Village

THROUGH MY OWN experience and by reaching out to experts in various fields of integrative medicine (those are the docs who treat the whole person in health—they don't wait for illness) and other specialists and mind-body experts, including nutritionists, physicians, and Ayurvedic medicine practitioners, I've come to the conclusion that, just like it takes a village to raise a child, it takes a variety of points of view to understand your body and create the mind-body connection that is so crucial to overall health, wellness, and self-care. What I do for myself is glean from these different sources. I've tried many approaches to wellness and discovered what works best for me. These suggestions might work for you as well. But really it's a process of trial and error because everyone is different, and you need to learn what works best for *you*.

Ayurveda, for example, combines conventional Western medicine with complementary treatments such as herbal medicine, yoga, and stress-reduction techniques—all in an effort to treat the whole person. (Proponents prefer the term *complementary* to emphasize the point that such treatments are used *with* mainstream medicine, not as replacements or alternatives.) Ayurveda teaches you to think of your whole person and that all areas of life impact your health. According to Ayurveda, molecules of negative or toxic emotion, such as anger, fear, sadness, jealousy, etc., are lipophilic, which means they take safe haven and store themselves in our fat cells, causing physical and emotional disturbances for years and years. When we burn our fat cells, we release these old patterns of behavior that we find ourselves repeating over and over again. Ayurveda is not a one-size-fits-all system. Instead, its regimens are tailored to each person's unique *prakruti* (Ayurvedic constitution), taking into account individual needs for nutrition, exercise, social interaction, and emotional sustenance. In other words, how we live affects every aspect of our bodies. For me, this is why Ayurvedic eating, which emphasizes whole foods that are alkaline, not acidic, makes so much sense.

From nutritionists I've learned the basics about what our bodies need in terms of lean protein, good fats (not the bad, such as trans fats), carbohydrates (again, the good, not the overly processed or heavily starchy), fiber, and all the wonderful antioxidants we get from veggies and fruits. I've learned why we need to take processed foods out of our diets, and to reduce refined sugar consumption to less than a teaspoon a day to avoid creating cravings and addiction-like relationships with sweet things. I've learned why many of us have developed intolerances to dairy and gluten. I've also learned how to make my diet more alkaline and less acidic. Highly acidic diets are associated with everything from weight gain and osteoporosis to irritable bowel syndrome (IBS) and Crohn's disease. Ever since I began eating foods with a high alkaline impact, my skin is clearer and I feel more energetic, and just plain lighter on my feet. (You will read all about these ideas and more in chapter 4.) I've incorporated all this varied information into a way of living that works for me, and I share it here so that you don't have to do the research but can trust that I have.

Ever since I began eating foods with a high alkaline impact, my skin is clearer and I feel more energetic, and just plain lighter on my feet.

I've taken the same deep-dive approach to exercise. My research in that arena, as you may have guessed, is to try everything! I move in a myriad of different ways, in different places, at different times of day, and for different amounts of time. I work to find ways of integrating exercise into my life seamlessly, or as seamlessly as possible. The same goes for how I approach meditation and mindfulness. And with clean eating, exercise, and meditation, you will learn what I do—but again, it's up to you to try lots of things, find what you enjoy, and decide what makes you feel satisfied and well.

Your Body Is Smart

OR ME, READING my body, paying attention to its signals and honoring its natural intelligence, is the key to staying slim, fit, and healthy.

If you want to lose weight and keep it off without deprivation or some crazy kind of eating regimen, then tuning in to your body will give you the power to take some control over your hunger, and get rid of cravings or the need for extremes—in terms of either food or exercise.

And that takes me to my next point. By truly connecting with yourself and accepting who you are and whatever shape you have, you reject perfection and the idea of extremes. From this vantage point, all of us can be happy—happy just being ourselves. Suddenly, instead of pushing against the grain, we give our bodies what they naturally need to stay centered and feel strong and agile. We don't have to force ourselves to eat a certain way or exercise a certain way. We work with the body, not against it. And you can trust that your body is smart and knows what it needs and doesn't need.

Thinking of my body in this way helps me not freak out if I've gained ten pounds (or seventy, like I did when I was pregnant with my son Ryder!). Because when I feel bad, I trust that I know how to get back on track. This kind of relationship with myself has not only helped me stay grounded and balanced in the midst of a very hectic career and being a mom of two young boys, but also has made me feel much more trusting of my body. I am so much more relaxed now, not needing to overthink what I eat, how much I eat, when I exercise, or what I do.

Not too long ago I would try to assert control over my body, pushing it way beyond what was good and healthy. I would work out to the point where I was exhausted. I would also eat raw and super-healthy, pushing my stress hormones through the roof because I put so much thought into every bite. In other words, if I gained weight, I tended to overcorrect and get so over-regimented and obsessed that I would either not lose the weight I wanted or sometimes gain weight. Then I would swing the other way and not work out at all. For example, I stopped dancing, an activity I loved, completely for a couple of years. When I eventually went back to it, I had to ask myself, "Why haven't I been doing this? I love to dance!"

Always trying to control everything around me and within me only made me want to break the rules. Think of a tiger in a zoo—sure, the tiger might seem happy in an almost natural, jungle-like confined space, but after a while, the wild animal inside will show its true nature. It will escape if given the chance, or attack if cornered. It may be still and seem to live for its next hit of raw meat. But we kind of know that underneath that behavior is its real wish: it wants to be free!

I'm not saying I'm a tiger at heart, but I definitely feel a kinship. I need space to run and the ability to wander; I need to feel my strength and flex my spirit. But I can't be that person if I feel at all caged in. I don't follow any steadfast rules about how I eat or get my exercise every single day. I am not an automaton. But it's through discipline that I found freedom.

It's Up to You

UNLIKE THE GENERATIONS that came before us, we are not waiting to get sick. We understand that our health is in our own hands and is an everyday, lifelong affair. So it's up to us to make good lifestyle choices. I must say, I learned this lesson early—from my parents, who, in many ways, were ahead of their time when it came to healthy living.

My parents, especially my mom, have always been enormously inspiring and influential role models. And it was from my mom that I learned to take responsibility for my body. I watched both my parents transform their bodies for their craft. Depending on the role, they had to puff up, slim down, add muscle, get lean. Their bodies were extensions of the characters they were playing.

But at the end of a project or film, they had to go back to their own Drawing Boards and restore their own inner balance, get back to the weight that was right for them, and get back to eating the foods they enjoyed and that made them feel healthy and energetic.

Observing my parents paying attention to their bodies in this way and taking responsibility for their health gave me a head start in knowing how to take care of my own body, and was how I learned that what I put into it had various effects. But eventually I learned that I couldn't just copy my parents. I figured out that it was up to me to take responsibility for myself. The older I got, as I would diet to lose weight and sometimes gain weight when I was (and wasn't) pregnant, I began to understand that the lack of control I was feeling was something that I was actually allowing to happen. I'm not being judgmental here or self-critical. I am simply making an observation about how I used to be. I had to learn—slowly—how to consciously make and then own my choices about how I ate and worked out, which I still do today. Sometimes I make good choices, sometimes not so good. It's still a process and it's always changing. And all of that's fine because I go back to my Drawing Board and take a second look at what I'm feeling, thinking about, and reacting to in my life. Then I figure out when I want to make new decisions or choices. I know I can always clean up my diet, change my workout routine, or restore sleep habits because my Drawing Board has the blueprint of what works best for me.

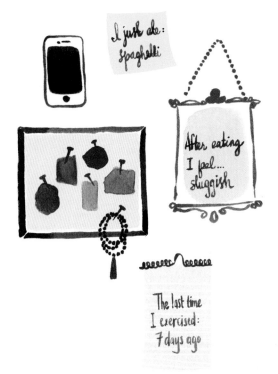

Your Drawing Board

THIS MAY SOUND hokey, New Age even. Maybe the concept of the Drawing Board sounds like a mood board or vision board to you. That's okay—whatever association you want to make is fine because you can create your own Drawing Board however you want.

Your Drawing Board is a place (or number of places) where you track your thoughts, feelings, questions, and fears. You write down what your body is doing and how you feel about that. You write down what your health goals are, or what you want to be able to do and share with your family. You can make lists. You can draw pictures. You can use Post-its and scatter them throughout your home.

I use a journal.

Your Drawing Board is a mirror of the inside of your head, heart, and body. It's a dynamic, ever-changing reflection of what's going on inside of you so you are aware of all of you.

DRAWING BOARD

Where are you right now?

We are at the beginning of a long and winding road. One way to get ready for what lies ahead is to think about where you are now, this very minute. First, on or in your Drawing Board, write down responses to the five prompts below.

I just ate _____

After eating, I felt _____

The last time I exercised was _____

The last time I had some quiet time to do nothing was _____

I was [place or location] _____

Next, respond to the prompts below to connect to how you are feeling emotionally and your awareness of yourself and your surroundings.

I am _____

I feel _____

I think _____

I wish _____

I hear _____

I smell _____

I fear _____

What's going on in your life? How would you describe your mood? Keep it simple, but try to be as clear and concrete as possible. This kind of tuning in to your physical body, your habits and how they make you feel, and your emotional life can help steer you in the direction of a more intuitive relationship with yourself.

Harmony Within

WITH A LOT of hard work and dedication in the last three years, I have finally found harmony. Before this time, I knew pieces of the puzzle but had not truly understood the whole picture. I was never an emotional eater, but I made bad choices about food or exercise sometimes. Now, after a lot of trial and error, I've figured out how not to overthink what I eat. I don't restrict myself. I use my Drawing Board to ground me, to reflect back all of what I'm doing and feeling so that if I feel off, I can make a few small adjustments. Because I know I am always changing. I've learned to enjoy new foods and new ways to be inside my body—and there are always new options to discover! And because I've experienced moments that felt like there was no light at the end of the tunnel but found support and got myself on the other side of some very challenging emotional struggles, I have learned to trust myself. There's no better feeling than realizing I have the power to get through the muck and the hard stuff to get to all that's good! This doesn't mean some of my old patterns or bad coping mechanisms won't crop up again—they will—but now I know I'm ready for them. In a way, writing this book is almost like a reminder to myself of how I learned to turn to nutrition, exercise, and meditation as a way to manage upheavals in my life—whether they are daily and routine or more complex and existential.

My Drawing Board has become my lifesaver, my safety net. It's the place where I can be brutally honest with myself. And as such, it enables me to always understand what is going on with me—why I decided to go off the rails for a few days, or why I feel so damn good, and everything in between. I hope that you can use your own Drawing Board to create that completely truthful relationship with yourself. It has worked wonders for me.

CHAPTER TWO

DIGGING IN AND GETTING READY

Is Something Holding You Back?

I T IS TIME to look inside yourself, to that place that has been the root of your negative self-esteem, self-doubt, and weight issues. Have you tried five, ten, or twenty different diets to help you lose unwanted pounds? Have you joined a gym with a plan to get in shape and then never set foot in the place again? Have you gained back pounds you worked so hard to lose, and then some? Have you tried and tried to change the way you eat, to no avail?

If any of these questions resonate with you, then know you are not alone. I've been there. It has taken me years to figure out the roots of my issues, and I am still in a constant phase of monitoring myself. Not in a self-conscious way that zaps my energy, but in a way that helps me keep aligned with how I want to live my life. Do I get off track? Yes. Do I wake up some days and not want to move or get out of bed? Of course. But this is why I rely on my four pillars—they keep me steady, they keep me going. Don't worry—I'll tell you what those four pillars are soon.

I'm going to show you how to connect with your best self, too—that place deep in your gut and in your heart that you know is there. Sometimes we have to get rid of our baggage and let go of negative routines and habits that keep us disconnected from our true self. In my past, if I was feeling drained, I'd withdraw, take to my bed like a Victorian lady with the vapors. If I had gained five or so pounds, I'd try to fast to lose the weight quickly. Of course, neither of these approaches did what they were supposed to do: make me feel better. But I believe we all have that good person inside of us who knows intuitively how to practice self-care.

I think it's important at the beginning of any journey to understand two things: where you are now and where you want to go. Your motivation and your ability to persevere despite obstacles is only going to hold and grow if you can be honest about these two points.

This is a huge part of taking responsibility for yourself and your actions during this journey to getting body smart. Remember those sound bites in the media and how they frustrated me? That's because these mini descriptions of what I do can never capture all the changes I've gone through. I've learned I have to embrace all the ups and downs, false starts, and backward slides in my life. I've gotten over heartache. I've also had to be honest and admit that my tendencies toward extremes—especially in terms of extreme exercising— either backfired or failed completely. These decisions and my past way of dealing with challenges and crises are part of my history, part of me—but I no longer let them hold me back. I've learned how to see that baggage for what it is—a part of my past that no longer works for me. But that doesn't mean those old feelings, old reactions to situations, and, more important, old behaviors don't surface—they do. I'm just much better equipped to deal with them now. If you've gone through heartbreak or lost a job and your confidence, you know what I am talking about. You may have found a new relationship or embraced your independence, but the wound might still hurt. Part of growth is taking the hurt and using it for something positive. This is part of happiness, but I also believe it is part of wellness.

Sure, it can be scary starting anything new—there is a fear of moving forward. Sometimes, it's a fear of leaving what's familiar. Sometimes, it's a fear of what lies ahead or the unknown. Sometimes fear makes us want to make excuses and place blame. Your imperfect parents. Your boyfriend or partner who left you. The job that didn't work out. Whether it's a fear or a tendency to blame, the result is the same: an inability to take responsibility for your part in the matter.

It's completely natural to fear change. Who doesn't? All change can be difficult, so it's important that you make big changes gradually. You need to identify your fears so they become concrete, and don't stay muddled and cloudy in your head. As I've mentioned, I thrive on change. But in the past, this was a more passive-aggressive relationship with change: It was more that I was running away from what I was doing—eating only raw foods, for example—to something different—drinking only green smoothies. I didn't sit still long enough to ask myself, "What's really going on? What do my body and my mind really need?" For me to truly embrace the difficulty or the challenge of something new, I had to become much more aware of why I wanted to change and for what specific reasons.

All things will and do change. What's important is to be *clear* as you pass through the process of change so that you don't stop or get stuck in a fear or blame cycle that throws you off course. What I've learned—and this was affirmed by numerous experts I spoke with—is that obstacles to weight loss and fitness have more to do with clearing away the emotional baggage than they do with diet and exercise. For me, working out has always helped me manage stress and deal with my emotions. But as I grew older, especially when I became a mom, I needed more than just a run or a bike ride. I needed to really pay attention to my body, watch what I ate, continue to stay active, and truly practice mindfulness. I needed to get clear. All four of these areas, these pillars, are essential to my well-being.

As you change the way you eat, add in regular activity, and incorporate even ten minutes of mindfulness almost every day, you will begin to gain the clarity and confidence to once and for all let go of the baggage that has been holding you back. The truth is this: I own my body. No one else. And it's up to you to own yours—your past, your present, and your future.

DRAWING BOARD

Without too much thinking, write down five fears that came to mind after you read pages 21–24.

1. _____
2. _____
3. _____
4. _____
5. _____

Now, look at those fears. Stare them in the face. How real are they? Why don't you try rating them? Do you think that if you lose weight, you'll still be unhappy? Are you afraid that if you look too closely at your life, you'll find that something's just not right? You may just discover that those fears are not as big and powerful as you thought. You might also discover that they are left over from a much younger, less wise you.

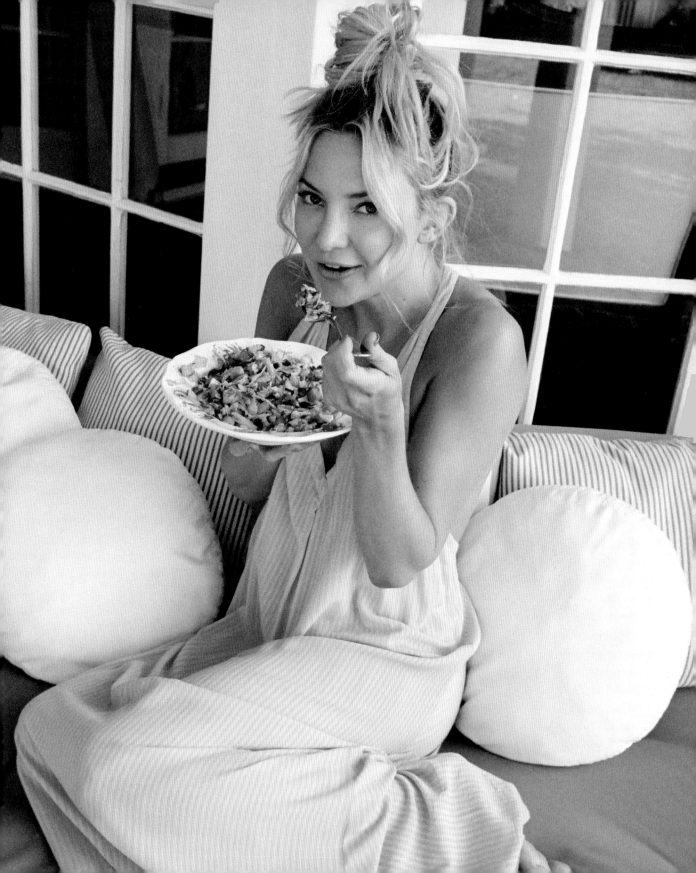

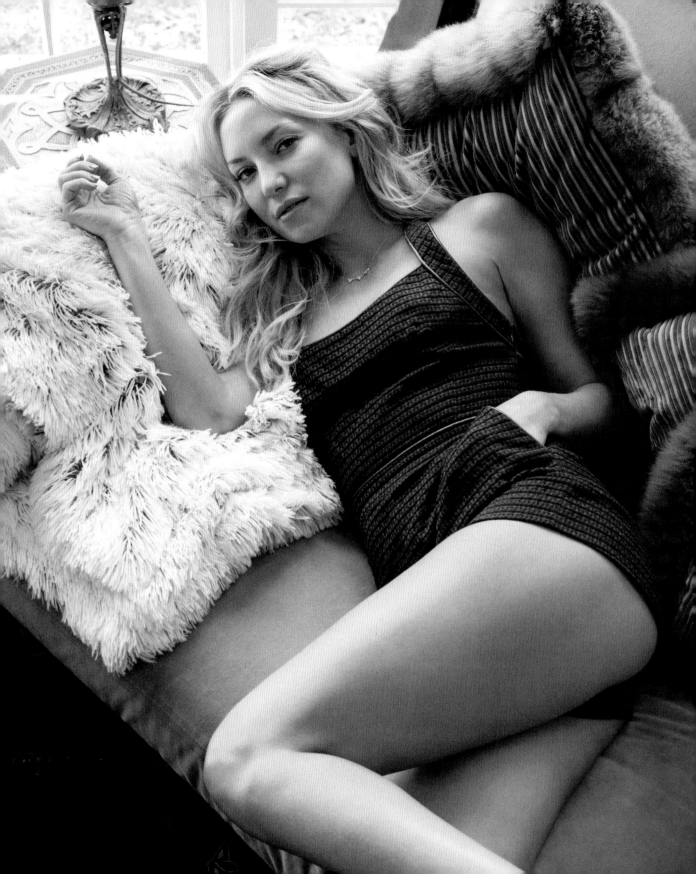

Your Four Pillars of Self-Care

AS I'VE TRIED to simplify what I do in my life so that I can share it with you, I identified four big actions that I use regularly to eat well, stay in shape, and stay connected to my mind and body. I call these my Four Pillars of Self-Care, and they just might help you on your own journey to wellness.

* Pillar One asks you to Cultivate an Intuitive Relationship with Your Body.

* Pillar Two shows you how to Eat Well.

* Pillar Three helps you Awaken Your Body with movement you love.

* Pillar Four will introduce you to the Miracle of Mindfulness.

Pillar One: Cultivate an Intuitive Relationship with Your Body. This pillar is your baseline. When you begin to pay attention to your body's signals and learn to interpret what it is telling you, you lay down the foundation for accessing and understanding your body's natural intelligence. Your body knows what it needs and what is not good for it. You will learn how to read the signs of health and the triggers that make you overeat or choose the wrong sorts of foods that never satisfy you, and why you loathe exercise.

Of course, there have been a lot of books promising to tell us how to achieve balance with mind, body, and spirit. But what I'm talking about is far simpler, yet incredibly powerful. What is my wish? That more women learn to honor themselves. When we make this a priority, we can find incredible strength—strength to overcome past obstacles, old stories of ourselves as less than, overweight, unfit, unhappy, undesirable. This journey does not mean the obstacles are going to disappear. No. Obstacles in our paths are as regular and reliable as the sun and moon rising. But you can get to a place within yourself that enables you to stay steady when problems arise. When you cultivate this knowing relationship with yourself, when you learn to listen to your body, give it what it needs, and take away what is interfering with its optimal functioning level, then you will be equipped to handle problems and disappointments without sacrificing your health and happiness. You will stay secure in your body and connected to yourself in a more confident, positive way.

Pillar Two: Eat Well. This pillar is all about the very real connection between what we put in our bodies and how those foods make us feel. Our bodies need nutrition—food and water. When you make good food choices, you will feel better and lose weight. These choices also reinforce that mind-body connection—the cleaner the foods, the stronger the signals between your mind and your body. Once you "clean out" the processed foods, the fatty and sugar-laden snacks, and the easy-to-grab carb bombs, you will feel in sync and energetic. Then if you occasionally indulge in something sweet, salty, or rich, your body's reaction will be quick and strong: you will know immediately that your body doesn't thrive on that food.

And you will indulge. I do. We all do. But there is no need to panic: You simply go back to your Drawing Board, take stock, reconnect with yourself and your goals and values, and then get back to eating well. Teaching your brain little tricks takes time. You're human. Don't get down on yourself.

Pillar Three: Awaken Your Body. This pillar is all about getting inside your body and figuring out how to be active in a way that is enjoyable and stimulating. Our bodies are designed to move. They are not designed to be sedentary. So many of our current health problems, including type 2 diabetes, obesity, and heart disease, can be tracked to a lifestyle in which people sit for long periods of the day without enough physical activity. I must admit: I have a leg up in this department. I can barely sit still. Exercising is something I do automatically, and when I can't exercise (if I'm on a long plane ride, for instance), I can go a bit bonkers. I will share with you all that I've learned from the many experts I've worked with and talked to—personal trainers, dancers, Pilates specialists, runners, and more—but mostly I will just share my own experience. More important, I will not tell you what to do. That is completely up to you. I will give you a variety of activities and routines that you can try, to discover what is enjoyable so that you actually *like* what you're doing when you exercise—that's solving half the motivation and discipline problem right there. It's absolutely key that you enjoy what you are doing. Being active is meant to be fun—like playing for grown-ups!

Pillar Four: The Miracle of Mindfulness. This simple action has changed my life. When I began to practice meditation and other easy forms of mindfulness, my entire body and my brain calmed down. I went from feeling up and down, like I existed on some kind of emotional roller coaster, to feeling in control. Which is not to say that I don't have deep, real emotions—I do, and plenty of them! Mindfulness does nothing to dull our sensations or our feelings. In fact, any kind of mindful practice makes you *more* aware of how you feel—but you are in control, as opposed to feeling like you are always in a state of reacting to your feelings. The idea of meditation sounds scary to some people, but I promise you, it is easy. And meditation and other techniques don't have to take that much time—just ten minutes a day is a good starting point!

Together, these Four Pillars of Self-Care will make you body smart. They will lead to weight loss and a better, firmer shape if that's what you desire. They will enable you to live harmoniously with yourself so that most of your days are spent feeling the joy and exhilaration of being alive, not bogged down, exhausted, and wishing you looked, felt, and were better. *Be better now!*

Contentment comes from simplifying your life.

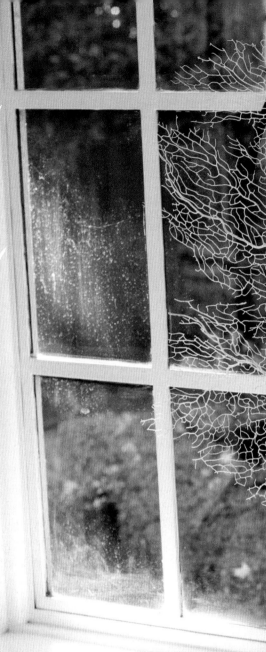
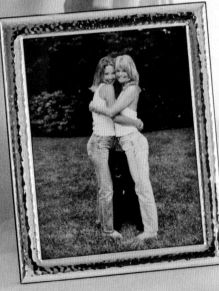
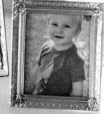

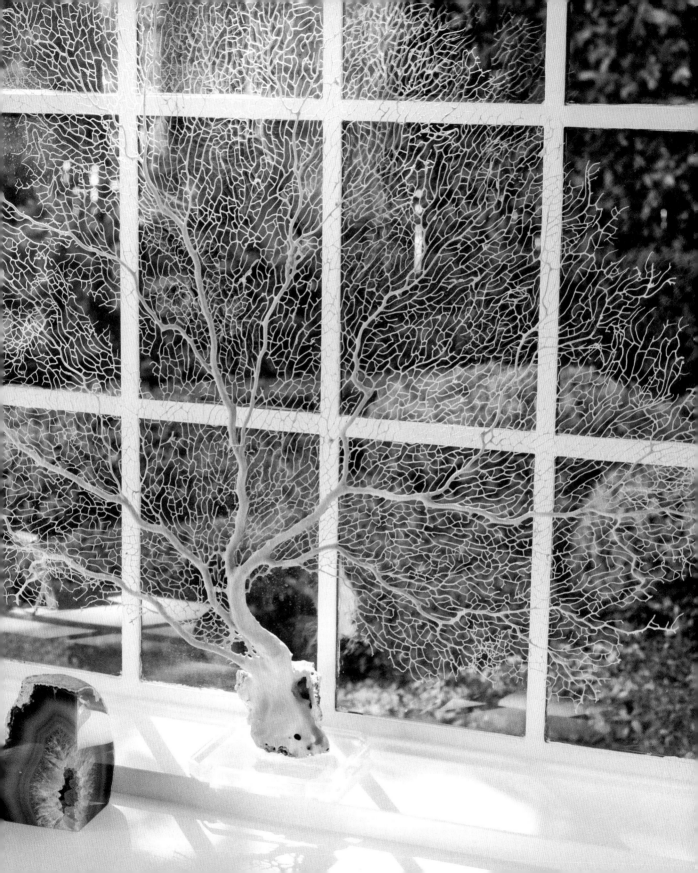

How Are You Feeling Now?

IRST THINGS FIRST. Before you can move on to the four pillars, you've got to check in with yourself on a few fronts.

* See if your basic physical and emotional needs are being met.

* Do a body scan to check on how your body is feeling.

* Respond to a series of questions to determine your "type," or, as Ayurvedics like to call it, your *dosha*.

This information, when pulled together, will help you cue in to where you are right this minute at the start of your journey—in your head and your body. Remember, you need to know where you are and where you want to go before you start.

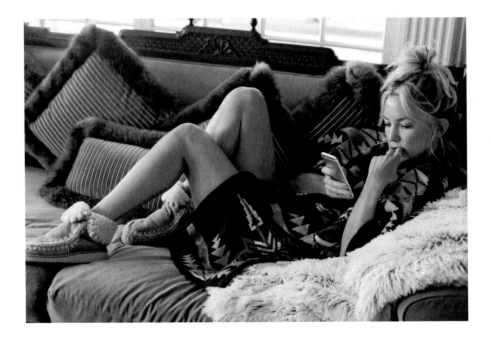

Are Your Needs Being Met?

I F SOME OF our basic life needs are not being met, then taking even baby steps to change the way we live will often feel too overwhelming. So indulge me and yourself for a minute by using your *Drawing Board* to jot down some responses to questions that are designed to see how you are doing.

1.   How would you describe the contents of your diet?

_____

_____

_____

_____

_____

_____

This may seem like too basic a question, but it's important to know what you are eating. We tend to eat mindlessly, getting stuck in patterns and not really considering all the choices we have when it comes to food. Really looking at what you are eating now will help you figure out what you want to change, and how.

This information, when pulled together, will help you cue in to where you are right this minute at the start of your journey—in your head and your body.

2. How much do you sleep at night and do you wake feeling rested?

_____

_____

_____

_____

_____

_____

This is another basic question. Have you ever wondered why there are so many television commercials that advertise sleep aids? Because more than 25 percent of us have trouble either falling asleep or staying asleep. If your sleep cycle is off, your body will be off. Its metabolism, its communication system (i.e., brain to body, body to brain) will not work efficiently, and your body will be in a semi–survival state with high cortisol, the stress hormone that wreaks havoc on our inflammatory response system—all these effects cause your body to hold on to extra calories and prevent weight loss.

3. Is your digestive system working properly? How many times a day do you go to the bathroom? Do you feel like this is too frequently or not often enough?

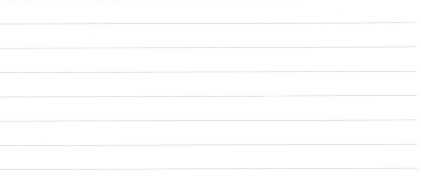

Your gut is everything. If you are either constipated or going too frequently, it's a sign that your body is not absorbing food adequately and/or is unable to get rid of waste effectively. Not to be too graphic here, but your gut is your single most important source of information about your overall health, especially as it relates to your diet. Learning how to balance the so-called ecosystem of your gut enables you to better process the food you eat (i.e., by taking in what your body needs and discarding what it doesn't). So, take note of your habits in this regard. If something's not right about what's coming out, something's not right about what's going in—or not going in.

4. Do you find it easy or strenuous to move and be active? How do you feel when you do something like walk up two flights of stairs? Walk on the beach? Run for ten minutes?

_____

_____

_____

_____

_____

_____

This question is getting at your overall physical fitness. If you bound out of bed in the morning, are able to touch your toes and run up the stairs and out of your house, that's awesome. If you feel out of breath when walking up stairs, if your joints are achy and you'd rather sit than stand, if even the thought of walking around a neighborhood block seems exhausting, then you have some work to do. Don't get me wrong. I am not a hard-ass who would yell at you and call you a quitter like some trainers, but I am honest: When you don't move, your bones, tendons, ligaments, muscles, and joints all begin to weaken and even deteriorate from lack of use.

5. Do you drink water or herbal tea regularly throughout the day? Take one day and keep track of what liquids you actually drink and in what quantities. Write it down below.

_____

_____

_____

_____

_____

_____

_____

_____

_____

_____

_____

_____

Is more than 50 percent of your beverage intake made up of soda, juice, or sugary or caffeinated drinks? Our bodies need water for proper digestion and overall functioning. Most "over the counter" drinks actually take away our bodies' hydration. Many sodas and other juice and energy drinks contain caffeine, which acts as a diuretic, making you urinate more frequently. In addition, some diet drinks contain a high amount of sodium, which draws water from your cells. In other words, these drinks dehydrate you. An important change I'm going to suggest is drinking more water and drinking little or no "processed" beverages. Are you peeing regularly? Is your pee dark and musty, or clear? If it's the former, then you might be dehydrated. Dehydration can cause a multitude of problems, beginning with hampering your digestion, making you feel tired and lethargic, and bringing you down overall.

————

6. Do you feel energetic and able to get things done most days? How did you feel when you woke up today? Yesterday?

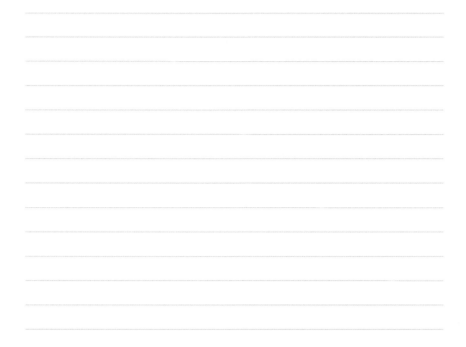

This question is related to your overall emotional-physical connection. When we wake with energy, it is in part related to our quality of sleep. But it's also related to how well or balanced we feel emotionally. I'm not a psychologist or therapist, but I will share some insights into how I deal with my own emotional experience—how I've learned to process confusing feelings and sort through what it is I am reacting negatively to when that happens. Our emotions are deeply tied to our energy levels and our ability to stay focused.

Now that you've jotted down your responses in your Drawing Board, refer back to them as you move through the book. Mark the date that you responded to the questions so as you move forward you can chart changes and notice where you tend to get stuck. You can also use this list of questions and responses as a way to choose one habit to change. Record all these notes in your Drawing Board.

Your Body Scan

ONE IMPORTANT ELEMENT of being body smart is accepting your body as it is, where it is, right now. Accepting your body means reconnecting with it—making sure you know what makes it feel good and what makes it hurt. You have to really be "in" your body in a very real, sensory-oriented way. You can connect with your body by using your five senses. This begins with staying in touch with how your body feels and what signals it is sending you. It means staying aware of how you think and feel about your body. Over the years, I have observed that those people who have the hardest time accepting their shape, their frame, or their physical characteristics are those who stay the most detached from their bodies. Before you move ahead, you have to give yourself time to be honest about the body you're in right now. Don't get caught up in an idealized image of yourself or someone you want to look like. People who are used to not liking their bodies tend to ignore what their bodies are telling them.

Here's a quick body-scan exercise using your five senses that will heighten your awareness of your body and make you feel more connected to your sensory system.

Let me be clear: this is not a meditation. This is a quick check-in with your body that takes only five to ten minutes. You do it in two parts: The first part is a relaxation exercise that helps you cue in to your body. The second part brings your attention to how those body parts feel.

Part One (3 to 4 minutes)

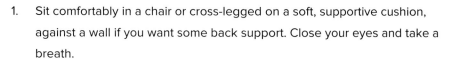

1. Sit comfortably in a chair or cross-legged on a soft, supportive cushion, against a wall if you want some back support. Close your eyes and take a breath.
2. Relax the muscles in your face.
3. Relax the muscles in your jaw.
4. Relax the muscles in your neck.
5. Breathe in a slow, relaxed manner, without effort.
6. Relax your shoulders.
7. Relax your back.
8. Think about moving your breath around your body, bringing it to your neck, back, and shoulders.
9. Relax your stomach muscles (without slouching over).
10. Relax your hips.
11. Relax your pelvis.
12. As you breathe in, bring awareness of your breath to your abdomen.
13. Relax your arms and hands.
14. Relax your ankles and feet.
15. Breathe in and out and think about the oxygen moving throughout your body, to your arms, to your hands, and then into your legs, ankles, and feet.

Part Two (2 to 3 minutes)

1. With your eyes still closed, go back to the areas of your body.
2. Does anything feel tight? Uncomfortable? Loose? Painful?
3. If anything feels negative in any way, try not to resist the feeling or push it away. Simply breathe into the discomfort and accept the feeling.
4. Gently open your eyes.

How do you feel? Are there any feelings or sensations you were not aware of before you did the exercise?

Now, go to your *Drawing Board* and record your feelings. What did the body scan feel like? Does your body feel the same as before the exercise, or different? Were you able to direct your breath to the various parts of your body? Were certain areas particularly uncomfortable? Were you surprised by where the discomfort came from? Don't judge or analyze what you write down. Simply record what you experienced.

The last time I exercised: 7 days ago

Your Body Type Questionnaire

ALTHOUGH I DON'T follow Ayurveda to the letter, this approach to overall health and well-being makes intuitive sense to me because of its emphasis on the necessity of the mind being in balance with the body. Ayurveda sees the body as a whole, and any illness is an expression of something in the mind-body being out of balance. For me, this way of thinking has helped me connect symptoms or signs, both positive and negative, with what I'm doing, eating, or avoiding. It offers some general guidelines to understanding our basic body type, personality tendencies, and the ways we tend to react psychologically and emotionally to situations and our environment. As you will see, Ayurvedic practitioners believe that there are three main mind-body types, or doshas—*Vata, Pitta,* and *Kapha*—though all of us contain aspects of all three. However, figuring out your general tendencies can help you begin the process of truly listening to your body's signals and paying attention to what might lie underneath.

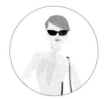

The **Vata** mind-body type relates to the elements of space and air. Their bodies tend to be thin and light, with a small frame even if they are tall. Vata facial features tend to be angular and narrow. Vatas like to move and change, and can be unpredictable—even to themselves. They are excitable and curious and can dive into the latest fads and fashions. They also tend to resist routine, so discipline and delayed gratification are often challenges. They like to do things on the spur of the moment and often resist planning, preferring to keep their options open. When they are in balance, Vatas are brimming with creative energy; when they are out of balance, they can be anxious, lose weight, and even have panic attacks. Their skin can get dry and they can become constipated.

Pitta's elements are fire and water. These types tend to have fiery personalities. Physically, they are usually medium in body type, with healthy hair, big eyes, and a strong digestive system. Their fieriness can make them willful, stubborn, and competitive, but Pittas like to get things done; they are known to be efficient and don't like to waste time. When Pittas are in balance, they are productive and passionate, and persevere in spite of obstacles. But when they are out of balance, they can become judgmental (of themselves and others), irritable, and angry. Their digestive system is where they become vulnerable first—so if they are out of balance, Pittas will suffer indigestion or a bout of IBS. If they eat foods that are too spicy (which they tend to enjoy due to their fiery personalities!) their skin may break out.

Kaphas are known for their larger body size, big bones, and tendency to gain weight. Their elements of earth and water are linked to being grounded and steady. They like to take their time and enjoy their routine, and they tend to resist change. People are drawn to Kaphas because of their steadiness, trustworthiness, and loyalty. When Kaphas are out of balance, however, they will eat too much and can be sluggish or sedentary (think couch potato), and slide toward depression.

Remember, all of us possess elements of all three doshas, and depending on our circumstances, our tendencies can shift. On pages 42–44, you'll find a common questionnaire that can help you decipher your main mind-body type.

YOUR DOSHA TYPE QUESTIONNAIRE

1. Describe your mental activity.

   ◯ (3) Quick mind, restless

   ◯ (2) Sharp intellect, aggressive

   ◯ (1) Calm, steady, stable

2. Describe your memory.

   ◯ (3) Strong short-term memory

   ◯ (2) Generally good memory

   ◯ (1) Strong long-term memory

3. Describe your thought patterns.

   ◯ (3) Constantly changing

   ◯ (2) Fairly steady

   ◯ (1) Steady, stable, fixed

4. Describe your concentration.

   ◯ (3) Short-term focused

   ◯ (2) Better than average mental concentration

   ◯ (1) Good ability for long-term focus

5. Describe your learning ability.

   ◯ (3) Quick grasp of new information

   ◯ (2) Medium to moderate grasp of new information

   ◯ (1) Slow to learn new things

6. Describe your dreams.

   ◯ (3) Fearful, flying, running, jumping

   ◯ (2) Angry, fiery, violent, adventurous

   ◯ (1) Water, calm, relationships, romance

7. Describe your sleep patterns.

   ◯ (3) Interrupted, light

   ◯ (2) Sound, medium

   ◯ (1) Sound, heavy, deep and long

8. Describe your speech.

   ◯ (3) Fast, will miss words

   ◯ (2) Fast, sharp, clear-cut

   ◯ (1) Slow, clear, sweet

9. Describe your voice.

   ◯ (3) High-pitched

   ◯ (2) Medium-pitched

   ◯ (1) Low-pitched

10. Describe your eating speed.

    ◯ (3) Quick

    ◯ (2) Medium

    ◯ (1) Slow

11. Describe your hunger level.

○ (3) Irregular

○ (2) Sharp, need food when hungry

○ (1) Can easily miss meals

12. Describe your food and drink preference.

○ (3) Warm

○ (2) Cold

○ (1) Dry and warm

13. Describe your attitude or behavior toward achieving goals.

○ (3) Variable or low

○ (2) Moderate

○ (1) Strong

14. Describe how you like to work.

○ (3) While supervised

○ (2) Alone

○ (1) In groups

15. Describe your relationships.

○ (3) Many casual

○ (2) Intense

○ (1) Long and deep

16. Describe your sex drive.

○ (3) Variable or low

○ (2) Moderate

○ (1) Strong

17. Describe your behavior in giving donations.

○ (3) Small amounts

○ (2) Nothing or infrequently

○ (1) Generously and regularly

18. Describe your weather preference.

○ (3) Averse to cold

○ (2) Averse to heat

○ (1) Averse to damp and cold

19. Describe your reaction to stress.

○ (3) React quickly with anxiety

○ (2) React moderately with anxiety

○ (1) Slow to react, rarely get anxious

20. Describe your financial behavior.

○ (3) Do not save, spend quickly

○ (2) Save, but big spender

○ (1) Save regularly and accumulate wealth

21. Describe your friendships.

○ (3) Tend to be short-term, make friends easily

○ (2) Tend to be a loner, friends related to occupation

○ (1) Tend to form long-lasting friendships

22. Describe your mood.

○ (3) Changes quickly

○ (2) Changes slowly

○ (1) Steady, stable

23. Describe your reaction to stress.

○ (3) Fear

○ (2) Anger

○ (1) Indifference

24. Which are you more sensitive to?

○ (3) My own feelings

○ (2) Not sensitive

○ (1) Feelings of others

25. When threatened, which do you tend to do?

○ (3) Run

○ (2) Fight

○ (1) Make peace

26. Describe your relationship with your partner.

○ (3) Clingy

○ (2) Jealous

○ (1) Secure

27. Describe how you express affection.

○ (3) With words

○ (2) With gifts

○ (1) With touch

28. When you're feeling hurt, what do you tend to do?

○ (3) Cry

○ (2) Argue

○ (1) Withdraw

29. Describe your common emotional trauma causes.

○ (3) Anxiety

○ (2) Denial

○ (1) Depression

30. Describe your general confidence level.

○ (3) Timid

○ (2) Outwardly confident

○ (1) Inner confidence

WHAT YOUR RESPONSES MEAN

Now, count up your points.

* If you scored between 30 and 49, you are generally Vata in body type and temperament.

* If you scored between 50 and 69, you are generally Pitta in body type and temperament.

* If you scored between 70 and 90, you are generally Kapha in body type and temperament.

Again, your score indicates your primary type. If, for example, you scored close to 49, you are a Vata with some tendency toward Pitta. If you scored 70, then you are a Kapha with some tendency toward Pitta. Go back to the descriptions of the three doshas (page 41) and consider your responses. Think about the questions and the ideas they point to regarding your behaviors, your ways of reacting emotionally and physically to stress and outside factors, and your quality of sleep, your dreams, and your thought patterns. All of this is valuable information as you move forward and begin to cultivate a closer relationship with yourself. Later, in chapter 3, you will be able to determine if you are out of balance (all doshas can be out of balance) and what you can do to bring yourself back into balanced health.

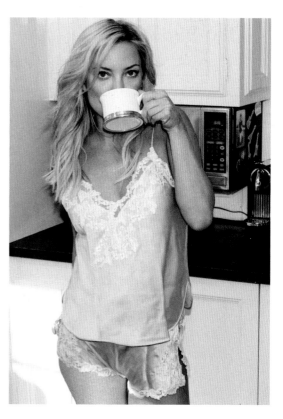

DRAWING BOARD:
MAKE SURE YOU RELAX

I know. Easier said than done. But every day we need to pause and make sure we have some downtime, to feel centered and grounded. This kind of touching base with ourselves in the form of relaxation is crucial to nurturing a positive relationship with our bodies.

I love to knit when I'm on set or at home hanging out with my boys. My mom taught me to knit when I was young and it's still my go-to relaxation method. I also love to read, do crossword puzzles, and cook.

We all know it's important to make time for ourselves so we can stay healthy. All work and no play makes us crazy, grouchy, and ultimately sick. So as you move forward with this process, take stock of the ways in which you like to relax and enjoy yourself.

1. List five ways you like to relax and that give you pleasure.

    _____

    _____

    _____

    _____

    _____

2. How long does each of these activities take? Fifteen minutes? Twenty? Five? Write that time allotment next to each activity.

3. Now, look at your weekly schedule. Where can you best fit in any one of these activities over the course of a week? Can you fit in at least three mini breaks each week for these relaxation activities? Write that appointment next to the activity, making a pact with yourself not to cancel!

4. Commit to this "me time"!

Be Gentle with Yourself

TO ALL OF us former and current yo-yo dieters, I want to pass along a little tough love. Along the path of change, it's human nature to lose motivation or sight of your goals and to stumble and fall. Do not take these moments to mean "I must not really want this. It's okay to give up." Or "I've already blown today. I might as well not try tomorrow." You must have a clear sense of what you want so that you won't question it.

It is also important to know *why* you are trying to make a lifestyle change. If you want to lose five, ten, or twenty pounds, fine. But it isn't just about the number on the scale. This kind of real change requires that you change the way you think. I'm going to give you lots of tricks to make it simple, but let me tell you—it's not easy. It's work and it takes discipline. That's why you've got to want it.

So right now, go to your Drawing Board and ask yourself what you really want. Try to make your goals crystal clear but also realistic. Do you want to lose two pounds or ten? Maybe five is a good number to go for in the first month. Once you reach that goal, you will feel more confident and trusting of yourself. You will build confidence in the idea that when you apply yourself you can take control and achieve what you want, and then you'll go back to the Drawing Board and change your goal to ten pounds. Along the way, if you plateau slightly or even gain back a few pounds, be easy on yourself. Forgive yourself. Go back to your Drawing Board, write down what you've been eating and doing, and see why the results changed. There's always a reason. Own it and keep going.

This is your life, your journey.

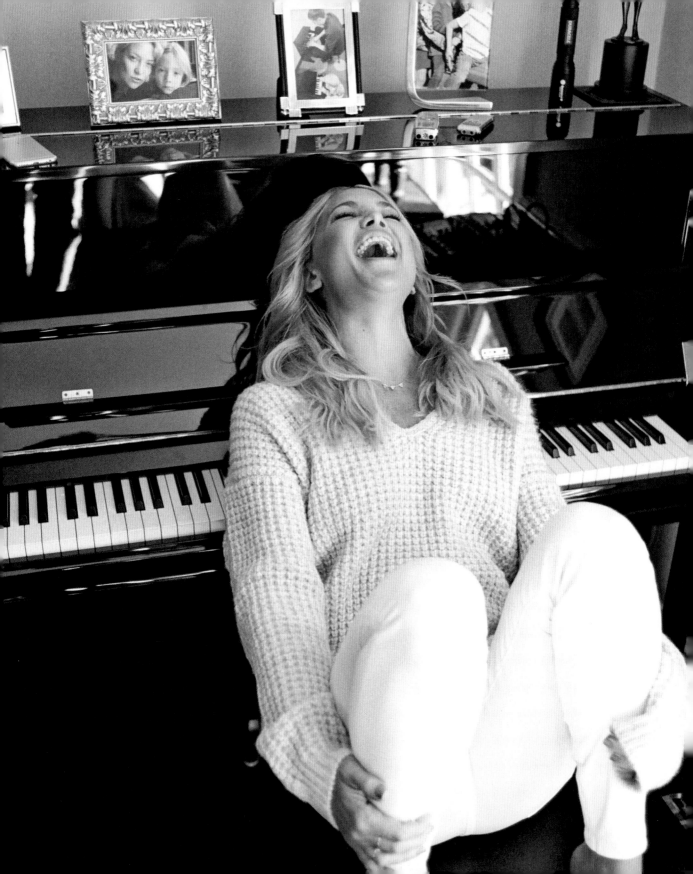

PART TWO

The FOUR PILLARS in PRACTICE

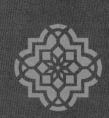

In the next four chapters, you will be diving into yourself. You will be using your Drawing Board for many activities and exercises to get to know yourself, your thoughts and feelings, your highs and lows, your questions and your fears. Keep your Drawing Board close by as you read—this will be an amazing source of comfort and reinforcement as you continue to nurture a closer relationship with yourself and change the way you eat and go about your day. This process, like this book, is meant to be interactive, so get ready!

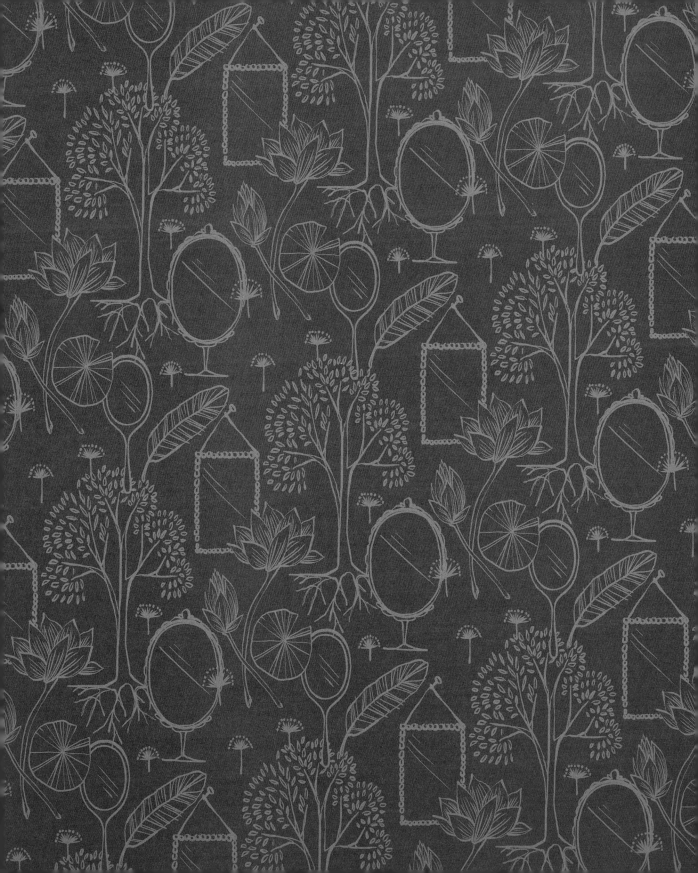

CHAPTER THREE

PILLAR ONE

Cultivate an Intuitive Relationship with Your Body

One Doughnut, Not Two

MY FIRST LESSON about food came from my mom. As I've told you, I'm a mover. As a kid, I never stopped moving: playing soccer, running, jumping, skipping—it didn't matter. I was in constant motion and spent as much time outside as possible. I also took dance lessons, following in my mom's literal footsteps. But when I was about thirteen, my body began to change. Seemingly overnight, I went from a scrawny kid to an almost-plump pre-adolescent. I was getting chunky, to be honest.

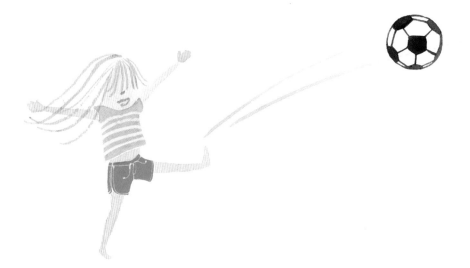

As much as I loved to move, I loved to eat. I was always first at the table and seemed to have an insatiable appetite. And even though my mom drank green juice and ate raw vegetables, my brothers and I ate "normal" food— breakfast burritos, pancakes and waffles, grilled cheese sandwiches, peanut butter and jelly sandwiches, burgers. There were Oreos and cornflakes in the cupboard. There was ice cream in the freezer. I didn't feel any restrictions or rules about what I should or should not eat.

One day after school, my mom casually asked me what I had eaten that day. Always one for supporting free choice, she didn't tell us what to eat. She wanted my brothers and me to think for ourselves.

Innocently I told her that I'd eaten two doughnuts, a blueberry bagel with cream cheese for a snack, and a chicken fillet sandwich for lunch.

"Two?" she asked casually. "Maybe just one would do. Doughnuts don't have a lot of nutrition, and your body is beginning to change."

Then she gently explained that if I started to pay attention to what and how much food I ate now (at thirteen), then I wouldn't have to worry so much later. I wouldn't develop bad habits around what I ate—and we all know how hard it is to break bad habits.

I didn't like the way I felt after all that fat, salt, and sugar; it wasn't about how I looked at that point. And while my mother wasn't suggesting that I was overweight, I knew she was right.

"Trust me," she said. And I did.

Of course, looking back, I think about those food choices I made as a kid—the doughnuts, bagels and cream cheese, ice cream, and fried anything—and I know now that they are trigger foods for me. They are for most people. The white starchy carbs that make me want to keep eating (and are so yummy) just leave me bloated and cranky after the high wears off, and inevitably lead to extra pounds. Though I may not have been born with my mom's super-slim, tiny body type, I wasn't born chunky.

> *The white starchy carbs that make me want to keep eating (and are so yummy) just leave me bloated and cranky after the high wears off, and inevitably lead to extra pounds.*

Yes—I am bigger boned than my mother, with more propensity for developing curves and muscles (from my Italian grandmother, to be sure), but my tendency toward carrying extra pounds on my frame was all about how I was eating.

From age sixteen to about twenty, everything seemed to smooth out. Then, in my midtwenties, right after Ryder was born, weight gain hit me again. During my pregnancy, I ate everything in sight. This continued when I was nursing. But once Ryder was a little older, I realized that I had not fine-tuned how to exercise in a way that matched the way I was eating. So I would gain weight and then put myself through hell trying to lose eight or fifteen pounds for a role. I'd eat raw. I'd try cutting out all carbs. I'd cut out all fat. I think I was just eating air. No, seriously. I tried every fad diet you can imagine in hopes that I could drop whatever amount of extra weight I thought I needed to lose.

This is what is known as fad dieting: going from one extreme to another in a way that your body *cannot* adjust to. Just like yo-yo dieting, fad dieting creates cravings, makes you feel like you have no control over your appetite, and basically reinforces all the bad habits you temporarily left behind. Soon you've created a cycle of restricting calories or certain types of foods, then "rewarding" yourself with sweets or fast foods or liquid sugar (more on that on page 174). As soon as you cave in and go back to normal eating, you gain weight again. When you drastically cut calories, your body reacts to the abrupt change. You start holding on to water, fat, and pounds because your body feels the threat of too little nourishment. Basically, any kind of diet that withholds certain food groups will make your body hold on to calories. That is how humans are hardwired. It's in our DNA. That is why diets work at first, but eventually they all stop working or plateau. This type of cycle can also be addictive, and undermines our ability to feel in sync with our bodies.

I'm hopeful that you can learn from my experience and take a look at your own habits and patterns.

FAKE FOOD

The one so-called food group that can be taken safely out of any person's diet is anything processed—any type of food that does not occur in nature. Take a look at the ingredients of the foods in your refrigerator, freezer, and cupboard. What words can't you pronounce? What ingredients are made of chemicals? If it's boxed and packaged, there is a high likelihood that it is filled with additives for flavor and preservatives to extend its shelf life. These are all toxins when they enter your body, have little or no nutritional value, and can't be absorbed. Eliminate one type of processed food—maybe chips or packaged baked goods like doughnuts. Take this food out of your cupboard and replace it with a snack of fruit—whole apples, watermelon chunks, or grapes. You won't feel deprived. You'll feel rewarded. Trust me.

You Gotta Be You

WE ARE ALL surrounded ("bombarded" might be a better word) by images of beautiful women—in films, on TV, in magazines, and in social media. The constant message transmitted by these images of idealized female bodies is that if you don't resemble, mimic, or strive for that standard, there is something wrong with you. We are made to feel inadequate and less than; even these "ideals" often have their imperfections pointed out in magazines. It isn't just men doing this—it is women, too. This onslaught of idealized body types in business and in the media is just plain bad for our self-image and gets in the way of accepting and owning our own bodies as they are.

Being held up as some ideal is just plain uncomfortable. Every woman deserves to be honored, not criticized or held to a bizarre standard of perfection.

Those of us in the public eye know this situation well. Our bodies are held under a microscope and peered at, scrutinized and assessed. It's not a secret that the media like to bring attention to how good models and actresses look only to jump on the first opportunity to point out their small or big changes and "imperfections." This happened to me most aggressively after my pregnancy with Ryder.

From the outside it looks like pure vanity, the hall of mirrors that is show business. But from the inside it's a horrible feeling to be picked apart in the press, to have your "flaws" described in all sorts of ways as a form of entertainment.

This kind of attention only reinforces self-critical and judgmental tendencies. The reality is, we all have a choice: we can live our own lives, by our own standards and values, or we can give in to what others think about us. Ultimately it's about accepting your body and not comparing yourself to others—myself included. It's also about honoring one another. We come in all different shapes and sizes. Every woman is subject to scrutiny—in the workplace, in public, in the media—but we have a choice. Do we succumb to the pressure and criticisms, or honor where we are in life and keep moving toward the next step?

This all relates back to self-acceptance. You must accept not just who you are at the beginning of this journey but who you were before and how you imagine your truest self in the future. You are all of those selves—it's up to you which version you want to emphasize.

All research to date on body image shows that women are much more critical of their appearance than men. According to the Centers for Disease Control and the National Eating Disorders Association, up to 80 percent of American women don't like what they see in the mirror, and more than half see a distorted image. Men looking in the mirror are more likely to be pleased or indifferent, or might even overestimate their attractiveness. Why? Women are judged on their appearance more than men are, and standards of female beauty are higher, more rigid, and getting more unrealistic every year.

The CDC and NEDA also report that women have an unhealthy obsession with thinness, and that starts as young as elementary school. In 1917, a physically "perfect" woman was described as 5 feet 4 inches tall and 140 pounds! Today, the average woman weighs 166 pounds and is 5 foot 4. In contrast, the average model weighs 107 pounds and is 5 foot 10 in height. Twenty-five years ago, the difference between the average woman and models was only 8 percent; now it is 23 percent. Which means the "ideal" woman is getting thinner and thinner and the average woman is actually becoming heavier. No wonder modern women are much more critical of themselves: only 5 percent of the female population can achieve the weight of today's models. This is crazy! It seems like we really need to ask different questions: Do I like my body? Do I feel good in my body? Do I feel healthy? Getting caught up in how we should look keeps us outside of ourselves and sets us up for nitpicking and comparing ourselves to others. What a waste of our precious energy!

If I could wish anything for young girls, it would be self-acceptance. I am not saying if you are overweight and possibly putting your health in jeopardy that you should stay that way. I am not saying that you should forget about highlights if you don't like your hair the way it is. And I am certainly not suggesting that you should skip the great outfit or not take care of your skin. I'm saying *learn to love you* exactly the way you are. The more you love yourself, the better you want to treat yourself and the more self-care you will lavish upon yourself. And here comes the age-old cliché: If you want to be beautiful, be beautiful on the inside. Let's hear it again and again.

So this is what I think we should all do:

* Respect our shapes and sizes.
* Embrace ourselves as we are.
* Nurture compassion for ourselves and others.

Only when we do this can we learn to love our bodies.

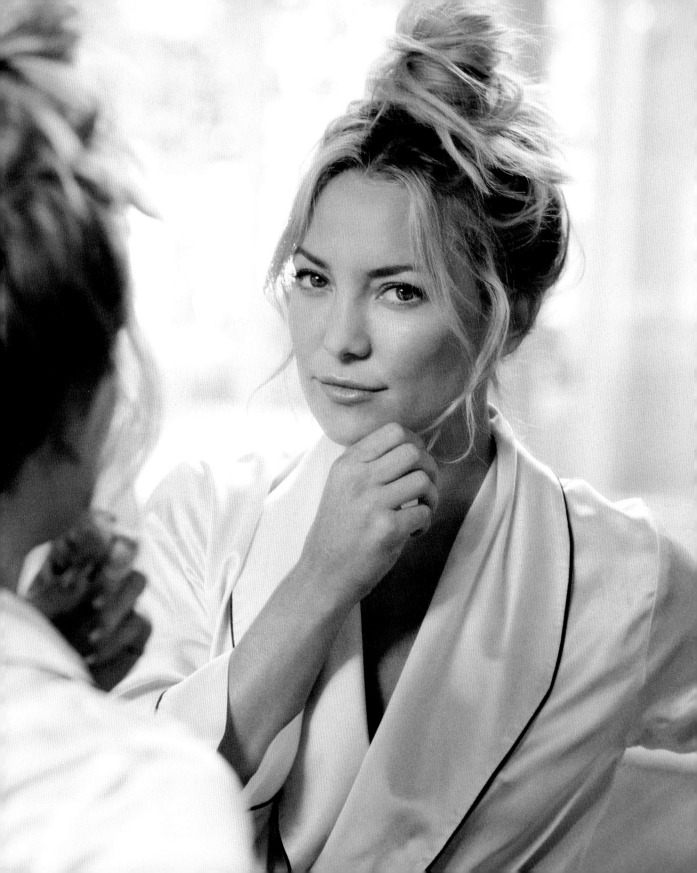

DRAWING BOARD:
LOOK IN THE MIRROR

Don't be afraid. Don't be shy. Part of being able to truly accept your body and embrace it, "flaws and all," is to really look at it. Step in front of the mirror wearing nothing but your favorite underwear or, if you are really brave, naked. Be honest and courageous. Now, what parts do you love? Your long neck? Those curvy thighs? Every part of you is beautiful! Write down what you see. Describe yourself—in detail. Write down what you see physically and what you feel emotionally as you do this work. Write down every word that comes into your head. Now, read back what you've written. Is every word that you've written down true?

It's crucial that you are able to see yourself honestly for who you are right at this moment in your life. You will begin to change—on the inside—and then your outward appearance will begin to adjust—but not until you accept yourself right now.

1. List five things you love about yourself.

_____

_____

_____

_____

_____

2. List five things you wish were different.

_____

_____

_____

_____

_____

The Trick Mirror

SOME PEOPLE WHO are having trouble accepting their bodies are, in truth, overly concerned with their bodies. It's almost an inverse of the detachment I described earlier. What we hear all the time from friends, family, and colleagues are comments like "I'm so fat" or "I can't believe my butt is so big" or "I hate the way I look in these jeans." I could go on and on, but I'm sure you get the picture. On one hand, these seem like every-day self-criticisms; no one ever seems satisfied with how they look. But here's the thing: these are typically people (men *and* women, by the way!) who are thin or in great shape! They seem to look in the mirror and see distortions of themselves. They are so blinded by their baggage and negative self-image that they literally cannot see straight! Psychiatrists call this phenomenon body dysmorphic disorder. It can be associated with eating disorders such as bulimia and anorexia, or it can exist on its own. However it manifests, it can be destructive.

Reframe Your Thoughts

YOUR BODY IS one thing, your brain is another. And they are intimately connected. When you reconnect with your body, you give yourself a concrete way to accept who and where you are now. And when you connect with your mind by staying in touch with how you think and feel about yourself, you give yourself an opportunity to know yourself on a deeper level.

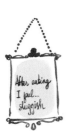

Go to your *Drawing Board* and ask yourself these questions. When you write your answers, be truly honest—that's the only way to really get in touch with what's going on in your mind. How do you think about yourself? What are your thought patterns? What does the internal voice that speaks to you usually say? What attitudes about yourself (and others) and personal beliefs shape your outlook on life? How do you describe your mind-set?

When we get busy in our lives, we can live on autopilot, unaware of our thoughts and numb to our emotions and physical experience. We fall into our routines, rushing from one activity to another, barely putting any focus on what our thoughts are actually telling us about ourselves. This happens to me on a regular basis. I have to remind myself to tune in, touch down, and do whatever I can to reframe where I am.

Both poets and scientists remind us that this thoughtless way of going about our lives breeds pain and discomfort and plants seeds of doubt. Day after day of not cuing in to what is swirling around in our minds makes us feel as if we are out of control, with no power over our lives.

But this is not true.

We can direct our thoughts. We can shift them from negative to positive. It's commonly accepted that when we harbor the negative, we get the negative. When we build the positive, we attract the positive.

These self-thoughts feed our emotions, which then affect our bodies—this is especially true of how we respond to stress. That's why the more we can listen to our thoughts and work to change them if they are overwhelmingly negative or self-critical, the better we feel. This is not just about surrounding ourselves with positive affirmations. This is about consciously training our thoughts.

Try this thought-monitoring exercise I learned.

1. Use your Drawing Board and take ten minutes to write down all the thoughts that come to mind about:

     ✳ Yourself
     ✳ Your partner
     ✳ Your family
     ✳ Your colleagues

2. Go through everything you have written and identify which of these thoughts are critical, judgmental or blaming, sad, or guilty.
3. Say out loud: "Wow, there is that negative thought about (me, Mom, etc.)."
4. Look at the thought again and try to identify where it actually comes from.
5. Ask yourself if the thought is true.
6. Take a deep breath.
7. Now, reframe the negative thought(s).

When I was a little girl, I used to tell myself stories—"I'm too tough, I'm not pretty, I'm ugly, I'm spoiled, I'm not talented"—on and on. It has taken me years to dislodge these false, negative beliefs about myself. But I had to do the work. For example, take the belief "I'm not pretty." When I traced the origin of this particular negative belief, I came to a familiar place—my older brother Oliver! He is only three years older than me, and I know that when he said things like "You're not even that pretty," it was because we shared a bathroom and he wanted his turn in front of the mirror.

My logical, adult self sees the innocence of the remark now, but if I hadn't actually traced it to its origin, I might still be reacting to that false belief. We all have false beliefs about ourselves that can wreak havoc on our emotions, particularly to how we respond to certain situations.

When you retrain your brain and dislodge these beliefs, you give yourself the chance to have a different perspective.

Think about a time a friend or someone at work made a passing comment about you being incompetent. Is it true?

"No, it's not true, but yes, I did not do my best work today." Your behavior might not have been as good as possible, but you, the person, are not incompetent. Separate the behavior from the person.

For the next week or so, go through this exercise once or twice a day, keeping a careful record of your thoughts. Again, don't judge yourself. Don't try to inhibit the thoughts. Write them down. Record them and go through the steps outlined on pages 63–64. At the end of the week, look back through the lists of thoughts and identify the patterns.

Who are you upset with? What exactly upsets you? What thoughts are no longer true or accurate? The more familiar you become with the patterns of your thinking, the more clearly you can trace them to their origin and the less they will interfere with your life.

This exercise helps you trust yourself. It helps you become more aware of beliefs that are false or true. And it sets up the foundation for the mindfulness practice that you will be engaging in for Pillar Four.

The Five Big Types of Negative Thinking

JUST TO PROVE to you that you are not alone, hundreds of books and thousands of articles have been written on negative thinking and how to turn it around. Why? Because as humans, we *all* get down in the dumps! In fact, there are official categories for all of the negative thoughts that flow through your head on a daily basis. So to sum it up: Welcome to the club. But just like training a muscle, we can train our minds to turn that negative talk into something that doesn't hurt us but actually helps us! According to cognitivetherapyguide.org, the five typical types of negative thoughts that bring us down are:

* **All-or-Nothing Thinking/Polarizing:** "I have to do everything perfectly because anything less than perfect is a failure." All-or-nothing thinking is by far the most common type of negative thinking. Living life has nothing to do with perfection, so when we set up situations to be all good or all bad, we also set ourselves up for failure—failure that makes us feel anxious, self-critical, and less than valuable. All-or-nothing thinking also gets in the way of trying new things—who'd want to risk that if they think failure means you're a bad, worthless person?

＊ **Disqualifying the Positives/Filtering:** "Life always feels like one disappointment after another." This kind of thinking comes from blocking out even the possibility of good things happening. Think of Eeyore: it's not always going to rain!

＊ **Negative Self-Labeling:** "I feel like a failure. I'm flawed. If people knew the real me, they wouldn't like me." How do you think of yourself? If you immediately label yourself using a derogatory or "less-than" term, you limit yourself from growing and from being who you really are.

＊ **Catastrophizing:** "If something is going to happen, it'll probably be the worst-case scenario." This type of negative talk is similar to disqualifying the positive: believing that only bad things are going to happen to you.

＊ **Personalizing:** "It's always my fault." When something bad occurs, you automatically blame yourself. For example, you hear that an evening out with friends is canceled, and you assume that the change in plans is because no one wanted to be around you.

OTHER COMMON TYPES OF NEGATIVE THINKING

＊ **Mind Reading:** "I bet she doesn't like me; I think she's laughing behind my back." We cannot read other people's thoughts, and making assumptions about what or how people think takes away our energy and our focus and tricks us into worrying about what others think.

＊ **"Should" Statements:** "People should be always be nice. If they aren't, then they are probably bad people." This kind of thinking is also a way we trick ourselves into setting up unrealistic expectations of others. When we stay centered in ourselves, we can resist trying to control how other people think and act.

* **Excessive Need for Approval:** "I can be happy only if I get all my work done/if my kids are happy and I am a perfect mother/if my boss smiles at me today." In other words, when we get stuck in a rut of constantly seeking approval or reassurance from others, we cannot feel satisfied with our own accomplishments.

* **Disqualifying the Present:** "I can't take a break—I will never finish this." When people stay either fixated on the past or are constantly looking to the future, they don't give themselves the space to really experience the present.

* **Dwelling on Pain:** "I'm way too disappointed; there's no way I can get over this." This line of thinking shows up when people are so tied to the unfortunate events or emotions in their lives that they'd rather stay stuck in pain than move on.

* **Pessimism:** "Life is meant to be hard. Joy, peace, and love are a pipe dream for idealists and children." Similar to all-or-nothing thinking, having a pessimistic outlook on life is based on the faulty belief that life has to be either all good or all bad, and that when we are confronted with a difficult time or painful situation, things won't change.

If you immediately label yourself using a derogatory or "less-than" term, you limit yourself from growing and from being who you really are.

DRAWING BOARD

Go through the different kinds of negative self-talk (pages 65–67) and determine which one you use, and how. Write it here:

_____

_____

Now, let's pivot and think about your strengths. What are your gifts and talents? Make a list right here:

_____

_____

_____

_____

Place a star next to each quality you want to make even stronger. What would it take to make that talent or gift even larger in your life? Say you wrote down *kind*—what a wonderful trait! How do you act on this kindness? What can you do every day to remind yourself of this trait?

Write down some ideas here:

_____

_____

_____

_____

_____

You get the picture. Knowing our strengths is one thing. Making them more present in our lives is another, much more powerful way to stay connected to them. And it should go without saying that when we honor these strengths, our flaws seem to magically become smaller. They cease to matter because we feel so full of ourselves (in a good way!).

Pay Attention to the Clues

TTUNING TO YOUR body means paying attention to your gut and learning to trust it. There is no irrelevant learning here: every detail can play a role in figuring out why you feel the way you do. Most of us have gut feelings about things, but we often disregard them. Or we ask other people what they think and we distract ourselves from what we already know. We all know lots of information about nutrition, good foods, bad foods, even when we are becoming intolerant to certain foods, sensitive to environmental toxins, or are developing an aversion or allergic reaction to certain foods. For example, if you started to gain weight when you reduced calories and all you were eating were yogurt smoothies, then you probably know your body is having trouble breaking down the dairy in the smoothies.

Following that clue is thinking for yourself and paying attention to what your body is doing. What I've gathered on pages 70–75 is a list of signs, according to the three doshas, that point to imbalances or symptoms and their likely causes. As you will note, some of the triggers for the symptoms are diet related, others are emotional or psychological, and some are effects from other symptoms. The information that follows will show you a few different things: first, it will help you identify your symptom; then to trace it back to its possible source. This can help you become accustomed to paying attention to your body's signals, and to figure out what's up and how to go back to your Drawing Board and correct it. This list is by no means meant to be taken as gospel, and it is in no way complete. But it could clue you in to what your body is telling you.

VATA

Vata is responsible for all bodily movements. If there's a disturbance in any of these bodily functions, Vata is usually involved. These include:

✳ Circulation

✳ Movement of food through the GI tract

✳ Movement of impulses through our nervous system

✳ Movement of thoughts through the mind

✳ Speech

✳ Communication

✳ Respiration (breathing)

✳ Sensory perception

Because of its mobile quality, Vata dosha is the easiest dosha to get out of balance, and thankfully it's also the easiest dosha to bring back into balance, once we determine the root cause of the imbalance and remove the cause.

The most common signs of an imbalance in your Vata dosha include:

✳ **Constipation, gas, bloating, or distention.** The primary seat of Vata in the body is in the colon, where its qualities function to absorb water and minerals from digested food and move waste out of the body.

✳ **Numbness or tingling.** Vata is closely linked to our nervous system, so when you experience numbness or tingling it's a sign of an imbalance in the nerve tissue.

✳ **Pain.** Pain is also signaled through the nervous system, including low back pain or sciatica and headaches.

✳ **Malabsorption.** If you have trouble absorbing nutrition from the foods you eat, you might actually have a deficiency of that nutrient in the body:

- If you have a fat deficiency, you may have light-colored, foul-smelling stools that are soft and bulky. Stools are difficult to flush and may float or stick to the sides of the toilet bowl.
- If you have a protein deficiency, you may experience fluid retention (edema), dry hair, or hair loss.
- If you have a sugar deficiency, you may have bloating, flatulence, or explosive diarrhea.
- If you have a vitamin deficiency, you may have anemia, malnutrition, low blood pressure, weight loss, and muscle wasting.

✳ **Insomnia.** Insomnia is another sign of imbalance in your Vata dosha. Trouble falling asleep or staying asleep typically indicates anxiety or difficulty managing stress, which are related to your Vata dosha.

Some major causes of a Vata imbalance include:

✳ Irregular schedule
✳ Eating old, leftover, dry, or raw food
✳ Not eating enough food
✳ Eating too rapidly
✳ Suppression of bodily urges, such as sneezing, passing gas, or elimination
✳ Staying up late
✳ Overstimulation of the senses
✳ Overexertion
✳ Excessive worry, fear, or loneliness

PITTA

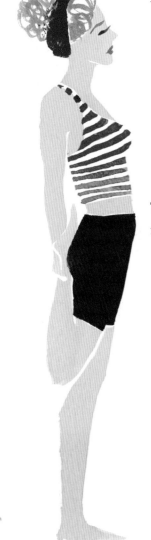

Pitta is responsible for:

* Digestion, absorption, and assimilation
* Metabolism
* Maintenance of body temperature
* Appetite and thirst
* Coloration
* Visual perception
* Cognition, reasoning, and understanding

The most common signs that your Pitta is out of balance include:

* **Heartburn, acid indigestion, nausea, or ulcers.**
  Pitta dosha is present in the acids of the stomach and small intestine. When these acids are high, it can lead to heartburn, acid indigestion, or nausea. If these acids are chronically high, they can actually break down the mucus lining of the stomach, which can lead to an ulcer. The best way to calm down Pitta in the upper GI tract is by avoiding overly hot, spicy, acidic, or fermented foods.

* **Inflammation, infection, redness, or bleeding.**
  Inflammatory conditions typically indicate that Pitta is high. Inflammation can occur in the skin, muscles, joints, or organs, and usually produce symptoms of redness, bleeding, or sharp/hot pain.

✳ **Skin rashes or conditions such as acne, psoriasis, or eczema**. When Pitta is high in the blood, it tries to leave the body through the skin, which can lead to various skin conditions.

✳ **Fever.** A fever is your body's first defense against infection. So in the beginning of a fever, it's usually good to let the fever burn away the toxins that are causing the infection. However, if a fever is prolonged, reduce it through the use of bitter substances, which cool the body while eliminating toxins.

✳ **Diarrhea.** The main seat of Pitta in the GI tract is the small intestine. When there is too much Pitta (digestive enzymes) being secreted in the small intestine, our stool tends to be loose. Again, the best way to calm down this type of Pitta is to avoid hot, spicy, fermented, or fried foods, and to take cooling herbs with meals.

✳ **Anemia.** Anemia is caused by the body's difficulty producing red blood cells.

If there's a disturbance in any of these functions, it may mean that your Pitta is out of balance. Some of the major causes of a Pitta imbalance include:

✳ Eating too much hot, spicy, or fried food
✳ Eating too much sour or fermented food
✳ Prolonged fasting
✳ Summer season
✳ Exposure to toxins, chemicals, or allergens

By the way, I'm a Pitta!

KAPHA

The functions of Kapha in our body include:

* Lubrication
* Growth
* Strength, stamina, and energy
* Production of mucus
* Support and stability
* Gaseous exchange in lungs
* Sleep
* Repair and regeneration

When your Kapha dosha is out of balance, some of the signs include:

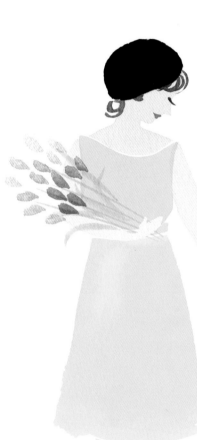

* **Weight gain or obesity.** This is the most obvious and prevalent symptom of a Kapha imbalance, and it's the result of slow, sluggish digestion.

* **Lethargy.** Lethargy is a result of the heavy, slow, and dull qualities of Kapha. One of the best ways to reduce this symptom is regular exercise.

* **Cold, congestion, or cough.** One of the main sites of Kapha is the lungs, in the form of mucus and pulmonary fluid. Because of

this, *pranayama*, or yogic breathing, is one of the best therapies for Kapha, because it helps to bring lightness and dryness to this part of the body.

✳ **Water retention, swelling, or edema.** When the body retains fluids, it's a sign that your Kapha is out of balance.

✳ **Increased cholesterol and triglycerides.** Excess Kapha in the blood can translate to a rise in cholesterol and triglycerides.

✳ **Diabetes.** Diabetes is considered a Kapha-type disease, often resulting from excessive consumption of sweets and/or improper functioning of the pancreas. There is a strong genetic component to this disease. People with a family history of diabetes may be able to prevent the disease by adopting a Kapha-pacifying diet and lifestyle.

✳ **Tumors.** Because one of Kapha's functions is growth, any irregular or excessive growth in the body, such as a benign tumor, is usually considered a Kapha imbalance. However, malignant tumors are usually considered a tridoshic (and more complicated) imbalance. Any kind of tumor requires consultation with your doctor.

Because Kapha is responsible for nourishment, anything that we can understand as an "excess" is usually an aggravation of Kapha (excess mucus, water retention, excess weight, etc.). An excessive lifestyle, as is common in the West, is the thing most responsible for an increase in Kapha. Some of the triggers that cause your Kapha dosha to get out of balance are:

✳ Excessively sweet, salty, sour, oily, or fatty foods
✳ Eating heavy meals, or overeating
✳ Excessive fluid intake, especially of cold drinks
✳ Excessive sleep
✳ Lack of exercise

ARE YOU HUNGRY OR LOOKING TO BE FILLED?

All of us eat for emotional reasons, whether we're happy with our weight or not. When you begin a gradual process of changing the way you think about your body, listening to its cues and honoring your feelings, you will reach for more whole, nutritious foods. You will eat more mindfully and stop reaching for food for comfort.

Ask yourself a tough question: What did you do the last time you felt sad, lonely, or scared?

Did you reach for chocolate or treat yourself to a Frappuccino? Did you indulge in a pint of ice cream or a sleeve of cookies? Believe me, I know how this feels. I am a particular fan of ice cream.

But when I began to truly listen to my body after I indulged in such high-sugar foods, I usually felt worse, not better.

The next time you feel uncomfortable, take a minute to let that emotion register as a sign from your body. Your body is working hard, so pay attention. Acknowledge the discomfort. Don't try to swat it away or deny it. Let it be.

Also, be patient, kind, and forgiving of yourself if you feel you've made a mistake that has caused you sadness, or if in your sadness you went for the comfort food. We are all so quick to blame and judge ourselves for just about anything, and then try to numb the feelings however we can. When we allow ourselves to feel our feelings, we are at much less risk of trying to cover them up with bad food choices.

Here's what you might want to do instead the next time you're faced with a situation when you might emotionally eat.

* Take a bath with lavender bath salts.
* Download three of your favorite movies or a new television series on Netflix and do a binge-watching session.
* Treat yourself to a massage or pedicure.
* Visit a museum or art gallery.
* Call a friend you haven't talked to in a while.
* Put your headphones on and take a long walk.

Your choices are limitless. The idea is to give yourself a positive, motivating distraction, one that gives you pleasure and feeds your senses.

In other words, reward instead of indulge, and remind yourself that you are trying to reset your body and mind. Push away old habits that keep you stuck in a lifestyle you no longer want or that no longer works for you.

Being gentle, kind, and forgiving of yourself is a very important part of nurturing an intuitive relationship with the body. You need to be able to listen with clarity, and trust that you will, most of the time, do the right thing.

Reclaiming Your Body

CREATING A POSITIVE relationship with yourself means honoring yourself, accepting your flaws, and recognizing your history. It means embracing your strengths and weaknesses and giving yourself a giant break so that you are not fighting against who and what you are. I also think this is part of the constant process that living this journey involves. I've had to reclaim my body not just once, but several times. When I first became

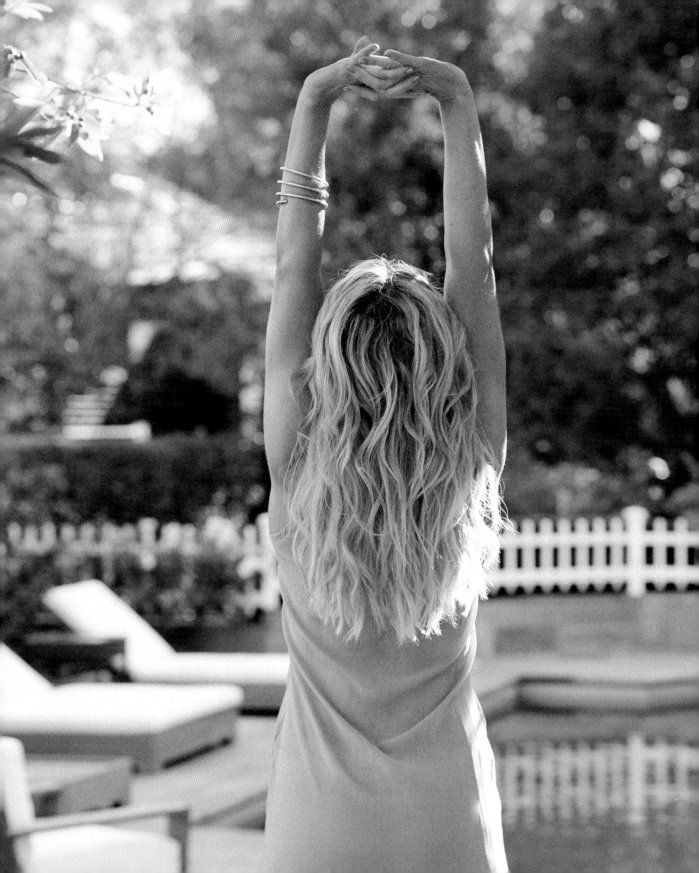

a mom, my world turned upside down. I was only twenty-three years old and had never experienced such joy, overwhelming emotion, and amazing love. Pregnant with Ryder, I was blissfully unaware of all that was happening to me and my tiny universe. As I've mentioned, I ate to my heart's content. I naively waddled around, waiting for my little bundle to arrive.

When his birth day finally came, however, I went through absolute shock. There was no way I could have predicted how much my life and body were going to change. In the months after he was born, I was in a bubble of bliss, caring for my son and marveling at the love I felt for him. But when Ryder was four and half months old, I knew I soon had to start filming for a new movie. As that time approached, reality started to set in. I got on the scale and saw that I had lost some of the seventy pounds I had gained, but not all. I felt heavy and awkward. This wasn't the body I had spent my whole life in! Yes, I had a beautiful new baby, but I wanted to reclaim my body too.

Under the guidance of someone I trusted, I started an athlete's regime of working out three times a day. It was intense, but I knew I had to kick up my metabolism, and this was a way to do it. For the three weeks that I was on this regime, I was all in. I was focused . . . and I was still a breastfeeding, emotional new mom dealing with hormones and a big life change. Well, my body didn't respond the way it was supposed to. And as the movie approached, the scale wasn't where I wanted it to be either. So what did I do? I started filming. I went back to exercising the way I always had. I decided to try to stop focusing so intensely on the weight and trust my body to do what I knew it could. And halfway through the movie, I was back in my pre-pregnancy jeans size. It was the stress and the pressure that I had putting on myself that was keeping the weight on. When I let go a little, the weight came off.

This is why it's so important to reclaim your body. I was pushed to do so by the birth of my child. But you don't have to wait for a big moment to reclaim your body.

DRAWING BOARD

Write each of these statements three times to commit them to your memory and soul.

1. I want to feel happy with my body!

    _____

    _____

    _____

    _____

2. I want to own my body and accept its shape!

    _____

    _____

    _____

3. I want to take control of how I eat so I can clean out the toxins and sludge!

    _____

    _____

    _____

4. I want to reset my body's intelligence system through whole foods and movement!

    _____

    _____

    _____

Now you're on your way to reclaiming your body!

Putting Yourself First

YOUR PATH TO self-care requires that you put yourself first. Plain and simple. If you don't put your needs, your desires, and your dreams first, then you will not succeed. For many, especially us parents, this may seem totally selfish. We are programmed to put our families first—our culture tells us that we need to sacrifice in order to show love. Not much in an average day is a life-or-death situation; other people and their needs are going to wait until you finish your exercise or meditation. Putting others before ourselves time and time again actually puts stress on our bodies and minds, and we may become ill. The irony is that when we take care of ourselves first, we are in a much stronger place to take care of those we love.

CHAPTER FOUR

PILLAR TWO

Eating Well

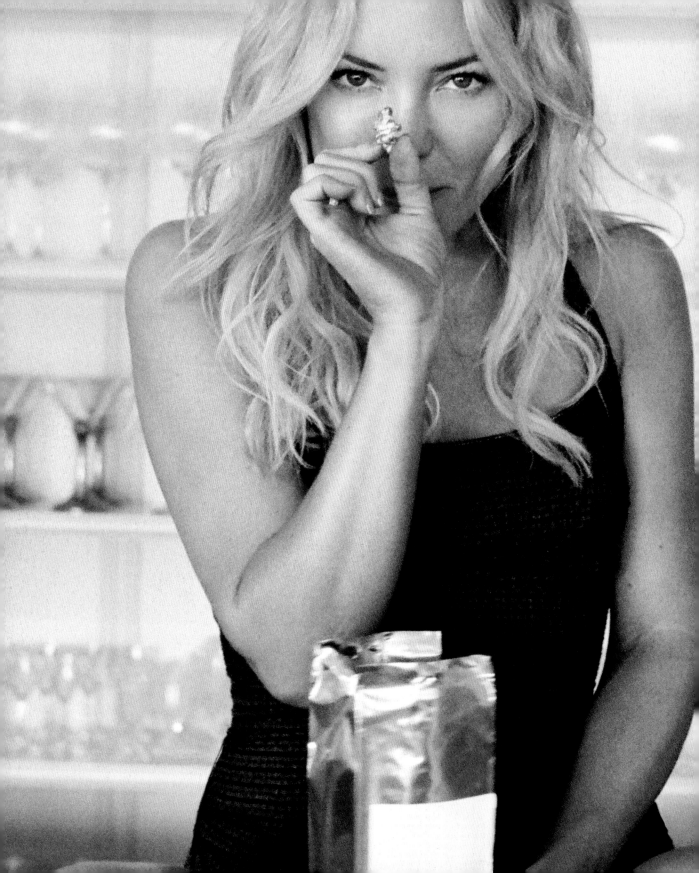

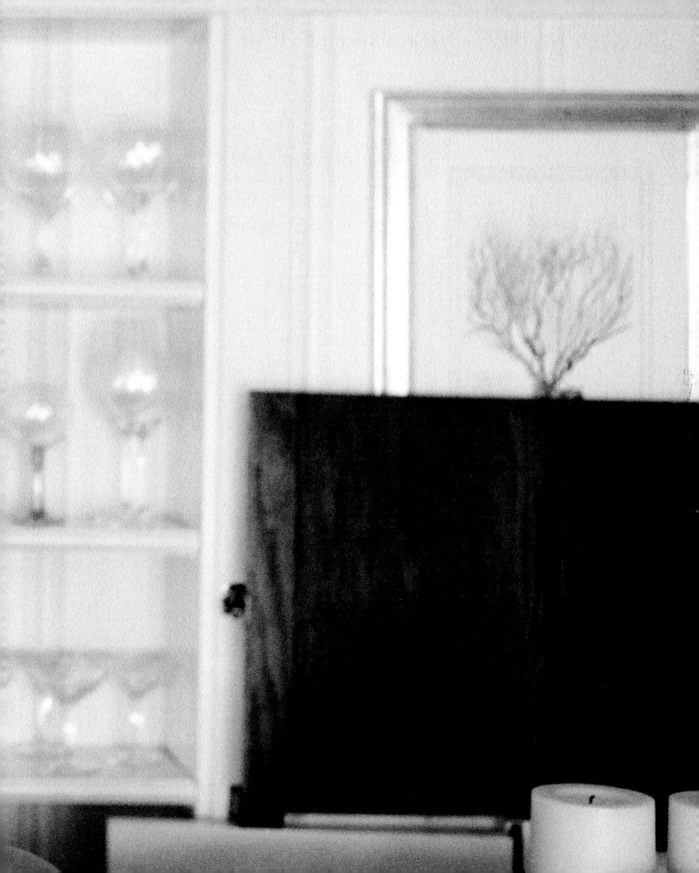

Riding the Roller Coaster

I T IS NO SECRET that processed foods and sugar affect mood and blood sugar, and make us gain weight. I had my own experience with this. I was one of those people who got caught up in the low-fat craze way back when. I would check out the labels in the grocery store, looking for foods labeled *low-fat* and *zero fat*. Of course, now we know that most of those low-fat foods contained tons of extra salt and sugar to create flavor, but back then, they seemed like the key to smart eating. I'd go for the breads, cookies, crackers, chips, all very processed no-fat foods stripped of nutritional content.

Luckily, I figured out pretty quickly that this was not the way to eat.

I've always been very active. During the no-fat years I was dancing, doing Pilates, and running almost ten miles a week. I skied during the winter and hiked whenever I could—basically I was in nonstop motion at all times. But eventually I noticed that I was tired a lot. Sometimes after eating, I'd want to nap. And despite how active I was, there was about fifteen pounds I couldn't lose.

On my mother's recommendation, I finally went to see a nutritionist, who reminded me of what I really already knew—that my no-fat diet wasn't doing my body any favors. It turns out my body was starving for nutrition! With her guidance, I cut out all the processed foods, including the crackers, the bread, the bagels. Then I added more vegetables and protein and fat.

This is when I finally started to understand how certain foods impact the body—the spikes in blood sugar that make you hungry and moody; acid-causing foods that make you feel irritable and lead to inflammation; how eating only one food group stops up the system. In the years since that time, I've learned a new way to eat. I've learned that food is meant to energize, heal, and build my body—and, most of all, I learned that I should enjoy eating!

Thanks to my mother's wise suggestion to see a nutritionist, I learned a few simple rules to keep me feeling good and my weight stable.

* Eat a variety of fresh fruits and vegetables with almost every meal or as a snack.
* Stay away from starchy carbs like white rice and bagels, and instead go for whole grains and legumes, such as lentils and beans, that contain more protein.
* Eat lean meat, but only occasionally—animal protein has a highly acidic effect on the body and causes inflammation.
* Avoid all processed foods like the plague.

Pretty simple, right? My Good Food List (page 101) will give you some background on the basic food groups so you'll know how to combine your choices for optimum nutrition. Use this list—along with my Grocery List (page 219)—to keep you on the right track when shopping for food and preparing meals.

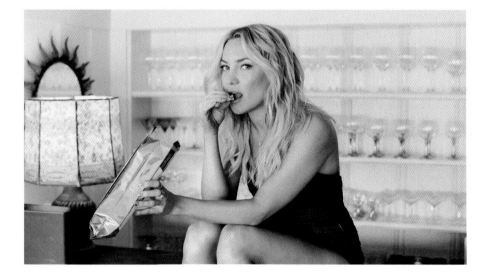

Change is my constant.

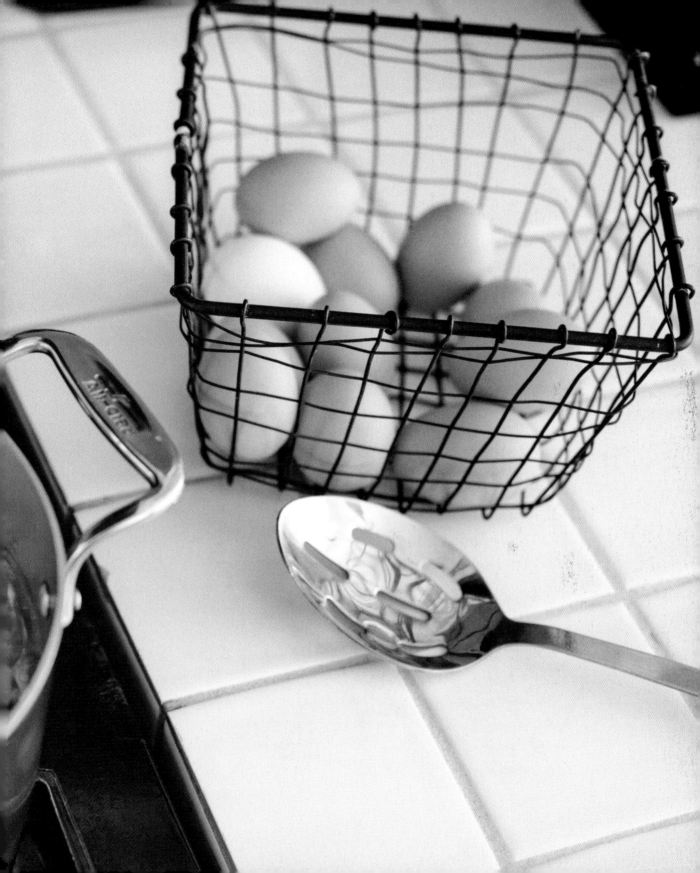

Restore Your Body's Balance

GOOD NUTRITION IS one of the most important factors in keeping your connection to your body clear and accurate. The cleaner and more whole (closer to its natural state) the food we eat is, the more our bodies work smart. On the other hand, the more we eat processed foods or foods that have an acidic effect on our digestive system and other organs, the more muddy our signals become. I know that when I travel or work a lot and go off my regular way of eating, I will feel either lethargic or jumpy, headachy, and irritable. My body gives me confusing, often contradictory signals, which is why even when I know I'm not making the best choices, I keep track of my food. This record—a short list I make every day on my smartphone or in my journal—helps me stay aware. My baseline for eating is actually quite simple: as many whole foods as possible. My approach is balanced, makes the most of high-nutrient foods, doesn't take too much planning, and will keep you satisfied—especially when you are active. It's a way of eating that is pleasurable and enjoyable. It offers variety—so you don't get sick of eating the same foods over and over—and the foods change with the seasons.

So many people begin a new diet or fitness program because they want to lose weight. You're about to learn that finding your ideal body is actually quite simple. It involves losing fat and gaining muscle. The changes you will make to your eating will be gradual, as will the changes that will happen to your body. Real change takes time. But I can promise you will lose weight if that is what you wish.

My approach is balanced, makes the most of high-nutrient foods, doesn't take too much planning, and will keep you satisfied—especially when you are active.

And since all of us are different—with varying starting points, physiques, and habits—in the way each of us responds to these changes in our relationship to our bodies (Pillar One) and what we eat (Pillar Two), we will all respond with slight differences. That said, as you make these gradual changes you can expect some amazing results if you eat this way. You can:

* ✳ Lose a significant percentage of your overall body fat
* ✳ Increase your muscle tone
* ✳ Decrease your daily stress
* ✳ Increase feelings of calm, clarity, and contentment

These changes to the way you eat actually build confidence and reinforce the intuitive relationship with your body that is so important to living from a place of acceptance, love, and joy. This is not New Age nonsense! When you clean out the bad stuff from your diet and replenish your body with what it needs and wants, your body restores its natural signals: you feel full and satisfied after eating, and you no longer experience the crazy ups and downs that come when the body is bombarded with junk.

At first, you might have to think twice about your food choices. You might have to go to your Drawing Board regularly and write down what you're eating so that you are truly conscious of what you're putting in your mouth. But I promise, after a few weeks of eating this way you will feel so comfortable that it won't take time or energy. (BTW, I will offer you some of my tips for how to make meal prep even easier so you always have your go-to foods ready!)

PROBIOTICS TO THE RESCUE

One of the ways the body takes in the nutrients it needs and gets rid of waste (toxins and food waste) is through the digestive system. An essential way to make sure the gut—the so-called brain of the digestive system—is functioning well is to make sure we have a healthy bacteria environment. That's where a good probiotic comes in! However, not all probiotics are the same. Ayurvedic health care practitioner Dr. John Douillard recommends that you take a careful look at the label and consider what imbalance you are trying to address. He suggests using different types of probiotics, which offer the body different kinds of support.

* *Lactobacillus helveticus* and *Bifidobacterium longum* boost mood and help the nervous system respond to stress, according to one study.
* *Lactobacillus reuteri* supports healthy bone density as well as optimal gut and immune health.
* *Aspergillus niger* is used to ferment sake and makes an enzyme called transglucosidase, which converts sugars into indigestible forms to feed other microbes.
* *Saccharomyces boulardii* supports a healthy immune response in the gut against toxins and bad microbial species.
* *Streptococcus salivarius* is found in the mouth and has been linked to a healthy immune response in the upper respiratory tract. Great for kids.
* *Lactobacillus acidophilus* supports healthy blood sugar, cellular reproduction, gut, immunity, and cholesterol levels.

✳ *Lactobacillus rhamnosus* supports healthy heart function, blood sugar, and immune health in the gut.

✳ *Lactobacillus paracasei* supports healthy liver function, blood sugar levels, and heart health, as well as optimal bowel function.

✳ *Bifidobacterium lactis* supports healthy microbial diversity in the elderly, optimal respiratory function, weight balancing, and blood sugar.

✳ *Bifidobacterium bifidum* supports healthy liver function, bowel function, and immunity.

✳ *Bifidobacterium longum* supports healthy cholesterol levels and bowel function, and provides protection for the intestinal tract.

✳ *Lactobacillus plantarum* (L.plantarum Lp-115) is shown by in-vitro studies to have excellent adhesion to the epithelial wall and to protect the gut from common pathogens. Isolated from plant material, this strain is abundantly present in lactic acid—found in fermented foods such as olives and sauerkraut.

Nutrition Redux

BEFORE YOU CAN make good food choices, it's important to know why you are choosing one food over another, and how to put together a meal or snack that is loaded with nutrition your body can use. In other words, there's no substitute for knowledge when it comes to learning how to eat intuitively. I've compiled for you a brief overview of the basics about food and nutrition—this will empower you to make the best choices, achieve your ideal body weight, and sustain this way of eating for a lifetime.

Your meals are based around macronutrients, the four essential compounds your body needs to function properly—proteins, carbohydrates, fats, and fiber. These components provide your body with essential calories for energy, metabolism, brain functioning, and growth. *Macro* simply refers to the fact that these nutrients form the basis of your meals.

Proteins are made up of amino acids that your body needs to build and maintain muscle, repair tissues, reproduce cells, maintain hormone function, and keep your immune system operating. Proteins are either "complete" or "incomplete." Complete proteins are those that contain all the essential amino acids (the building blocks of proteins). These proteins are high in quality and are easily absorbed by our bodies: egg whites are considered the highest-quality protein; other complete proteins include fish, chicken, turkey, lean beef, low-fat hard cheese, tofu, and whey or soy protein powder.

Incomplete proteins are plant proteins that lack one or more of the essential amino acids; they include beans and legumes, nuts, and some whole grains. Combining plant proteins is a good way to get dense, nutritious protein at every meal.

Carbohydrates are your body's primary fuel and energy source. Your muscles need carbs to function, as do your brain and central nervous system. Remember my low-fat diet that left me feeling so fatigued? When I took out the carbs, I had no energy! Carbs break down into good sugars (glucose and glycogen) that your body then converts into usable energy. When your body gets the right carbs, your blood sugar stabilizes, you feel balanced—not hungry—and you maintain steady energy levels throughout the day (though you will see that it's important to eat frequently so that your energy doesn't dip and trigger a not-so-good choice!).

Sources of good carbs include vegetables, fruits, whole grains, small amounts of certain kinds of pasta, and some dairy products. The best carbs also contain high amounts of fiber, which slows down digestion and allows the body to take in enough nutrition to produce the energy it needs without driving up glucose levels. For example, rice is starchy carb, but whole-grain rice (i.e., brown rice) contains more fiber and has less of an impact on blood sugar.

Packaged carbs such as crackers, cookies, store-bought breads, and enriched white rice and pasta all contain less fiber and more sugar. These types of carbs send your blood sugar spiking, cause a quick crash of energy after the initial surge, and have less nutritional value.

SUGAR AND YOUR SYSTEM

The body has two primary sources of energy: fat and sugar. All carbohydrates turn into sugar when they're broken down in the digestive system. This sugar converts first into glucose and then into glycogen and is either used by your muscles or stored as fat. In other words, if your muscles don't use up the glycogen, it converts into fat. This is one of the main causes of type 2 diabetes: too much sugar in the blood causes an increase in both the insulin release and fat storage. The body simply can't break down all the sugar and use it as fuel. This is one of the reasons low-carb diets became so popular; when the body has fewer carbs in the diet, it burns its fat stores for energy. Unfortunately, the body needs carbs for energy; when it relies only on fat, it sets off a negative chemical reaction that eventually creates a highly acidic environment in the gut and makes us sick. Our bodies are meant to run on ingested high-quality carbs that contain fiber, some lean protein, and good fat. It's the well-rounded, rich variety of foods that the body responds to best and that help to restore its natural harmony.

Micronutrients are the vitamins, minerals, and trace elements found in foods or taken in supplement form. Unfortunately, since much of our soil is depleted of these naturally occurring vitamins and minerals, unless you are eating organic foods from local farms, it's a good idea to supplement your diet with a great multivitamin.

———

The Four Rules of Eating Well

L OSING FAT AND arriving at your ideal body weight is not about deprivation; it is about creating healthy habits that you can realistically live with forever.

My approach to eating well is made up of four simple rules:

1. Choose well.
2. Control your portions.
3. Eat often.
4. Eat the right combination of foods.

When you combine these four rules with even a moderate level of physical activity, you will begin to lose fat and gain muscle. You might not see a big difference on the scale, but trust that your body composition is changing and you will look leaner and feel lighter.

CHOOSE WELL

Simple whole foods are your ticket to a great body, inside and out. Fruits, vegetables, and whole grains can be found in abundance wherever you live these days, and these foods should become the foundation of all your snacks and meals. When you subtract processed foods from your diet and replace them with whole foods (foods that occur in nature), your meals will be nutrient dense and much more satisfying. Processed foods not only contain dangerous additives and are high in calories but also don't offer our bodies usable nutrition. So we eat more and rarely feel satisfied. Although our bodies need the four basic nutrient groups (protein, carbohydrates, fats, and fiber), the sources for these choices are important. Think about these four guidelines to choosing well:

———

✳ **Eat a variety of foods.** Choose vegetables and fruits of many colors. A colorful diet is also a well-balanced diet high in vitamins and minerals and fiber. Take a look in your fridge: Do you see a lot of color? Do you see fresh fruits and veggies? Variety also applies to your choice of proteins—don't rely only on beef or chicken. Vary your protein choices to include lamb, turkey, tofu, beans, and legumes.

✳ **Eat seasonally and locally.** You may have noticed a growing trend to eat locally and seasonally—and not just in California, where I live. It's now possible to find farmers' markets or fresh food markets in most cities and towns around the country. When you eat with the seasons and choose fruits and vegetables that don't travel great distances, you will find more nutritious foods with fewer pesticides and preservatives.

✳ **Pile on the vegetables.** Your plate should be made up primarily of vegetables. Americans have a tendency to be "meat forward." That is, they make the meat or protein the feature of any meal. If you feature vegetables and grains instead, you will eat much more fiber, fill up more quickly on the most nutrient-rich choices, and can still enjoy fish, poultry, or red meat.

✳ **Drink your water.** Our bodies need at least eight to ten glasses of water a day. We've all heard this a million times, and yet so many of us still don't get our water in. The eight to ten glasses include herbal tea or flavored water. You want to avoid soda, energy drinks, sugary beverages, and other "flavor-enhanced" potions. Per the CDC, keep alcohol consumption to a minimum—one drink per day for women and two drinks per day for men is considered moderate. In combination with fresh, whole foods, plenty of water will make you feel satiated and energized.

THE BELLY FAT PROBLEM

High levels of cortisol—the hormone our bodies release when we experience stress—have been shown to contribute to a higher level of fat in the body, especially deep belly fat. Many factors can lift your levels of cortisol—chronic stress, lack of sleep, smoking, and drinking alcohol excessively, to name a few. Essentially the brain perceives many emotional and physical stimuli as stressful, and when our bodies are flooded with cortisol day in and day out, we hold on to fat in self-preservation—a hangover from our prehistoric survival wiring. The good news is, you can get rid of this deep belly fat by following three steps: control your portions; eat a combination of protein, good carbs, and healthy fat in each meal; and exercise! Over time (four to six weeks), your body will "use" up the stored fat and you will lose weight.

CONTROL YOUR PORTIONS

Although I sometimes count calories just to see what the numbers are on a certain food (a slice of pizza, for instance), I typically just watch the size of my portions. You don't have to use a calculator or a measuring cup at every meal. You just get used to eyeballing how much of any food will make you feel satisfied. It goes without saying that portion sizes at many "casual restaurants" in this country are out of control—from supersized sodas to value meals. Americans have created an obesity epidemic in one generation, with millions addicted to processed foods, which are cheap, plentiful, and ubiquitous.

So as a rule of thumb, think of these "eyeball" portion guides as a way to stop mindlessly eating when you are way past your hunger point.

✳ Protein: size of the palm of your hand

✳ Starchy carbs (like rice, pasta, or potatoes): size of your fist

✳ Whole grains: size of two fists

✳ Fruits and vegetables: size of two palms

✳ Fats (such as olive oil, avocado, or peanut butter): size of two thumbs

A quick note on portion control and food combination: in reality, there is no limit to the amount of veggies you can enjoy; they are loaded with fiber and vitamins and help you feel full (satiated) and assist in getting rid of waste from your body. However, if you're really going for that loss of 7 percent body fat and really trying to lose five to ten pounds, then use these portion size recommendations to help you eat a moderate amount of food at each meal and snack.

EAT FREQUENTLY

There's been a lot of controversy out there lately about how frequently to eat. Classic diet advice is to eat only three meals a day, but more current nutritional guidelines recommend that we eat five times a day—three meals with two healthy snacks in between—to maintain proper blood sugar balance. So here is my normal eating schedule, based on what I've learned.

✳ Eat breakfast within thirty minutes of waking.

✳ Eat every four hours, and include three meals and at least two snacks.

✳ Choose a time—at least two hours before bed—to stop eating for the day.

That last piece of advice is to curb the habit that many of us indulge in—mindless eating while watching TV, reading, or perusing the Internet or social media. Some days we feel more or less hungry than others. Sometimes this is because of what we are doing or the foods we ate the day before. But if you stick to your regular portion sizes and the timing of your meals, then you avoid triggering any kind of out-of-control or binge eating.

COMBINE YOUR FOODS SO THEY DELIVER

This rule is also basic, but I think it's worth pointing out: every meal should contain a combination of protein, carbs, fiber, and fat. This combination is not just so your body gets sufficient nutrition: the combination itself is the most satisfying and satiating. If your body is full, you feel satisfied, and you are much less likely to overeat. Mindless eating undermines the brain's signal to the body that it's full. (Check out the Good Food List on the next page to help you decide what's good and not so good for you.)

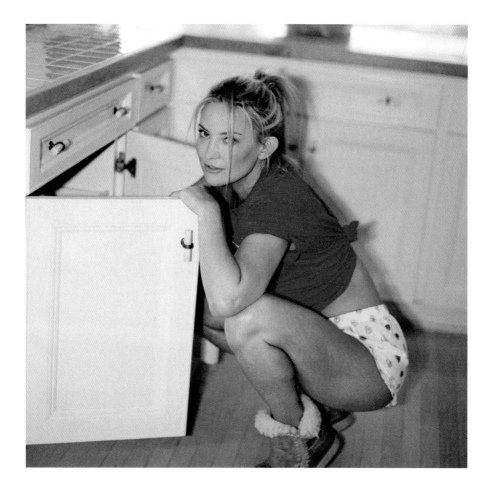

GOOD FOOD LIST

GOOD CARBS

Artichokes

Asparagus

Broccoli

Brussels sprouts

Cabbage

Cauliflower

Celery

Collard greens

Cucumbers

Eggplants

Green beans

Lettuces

Onions

Peppers

Snow peas

Spinach

Sprouts

Tomatoes

Turnips

Yellow squash

Zucchini

FRUITS (SIMPLE CARBS)

Apples

Blackberries

Blueberries

Cantaloupe

Cherries

Coconuts

Figs

Grapefruits

Kiwis

Lemons

Limes

Oranges

Peaches

Pears

Plums

Pomegranates

Raspberries

Strawberries

WHOLE GRAINS

Barley

Brown or wild rice

Bulgur

Multigrain cereal (or steel-cut oatmeal)

Quinoa

Sweet potatoes

Whole-grain bread (Ezekiel 4:9 brand, or bread with more than 6 grams of fiber per slice)

BREADS AND CRACKERS

Sprouted wheat

Whole-grain pita

PROTEINS

Abalone

Beef tenderloin*

Buffalo

Calamari

Chicken breast*

*Indicates foods that have a highly acidic effect on the body; for more on the harmful effects of highly acidic foods, see page 105.

Cod

Cornish hens

Crab

Haddock

Halibut

Lean ground beef*

Lean ground turkey

Lobster

Mackerel

Oysters, mussels, clams

Pork tenderloin*

Prawns

Salmon

Scallops

Sea bass

Shrimp

Sirloin*

Snapper

Tuna

Turkey breast*

Veal chop

PROTEIN—DAIRY

Cottage cheese

Egg whites

Feta

Low-fat cheese

Parmesan

Provolone

LEGUMES

Beans

Lentils

Tofu

PROTEIN POWDERS

Egg whites

Soy

Whey

FATS

Almonds

Brazil nuts

Cashews

Oils: coconut, flax, olive, peanut, soy-bean, walnut

Peanut butter

Peanuts

Pistachios

Walnuts

*Indicates foods that have a highly acidic effect on the body; for more on the harmful effects of highly acidic foods, see page 105.

This combination is not just so your body gets sufficient nutrition: the combination itself is the most satisfying and satiating.

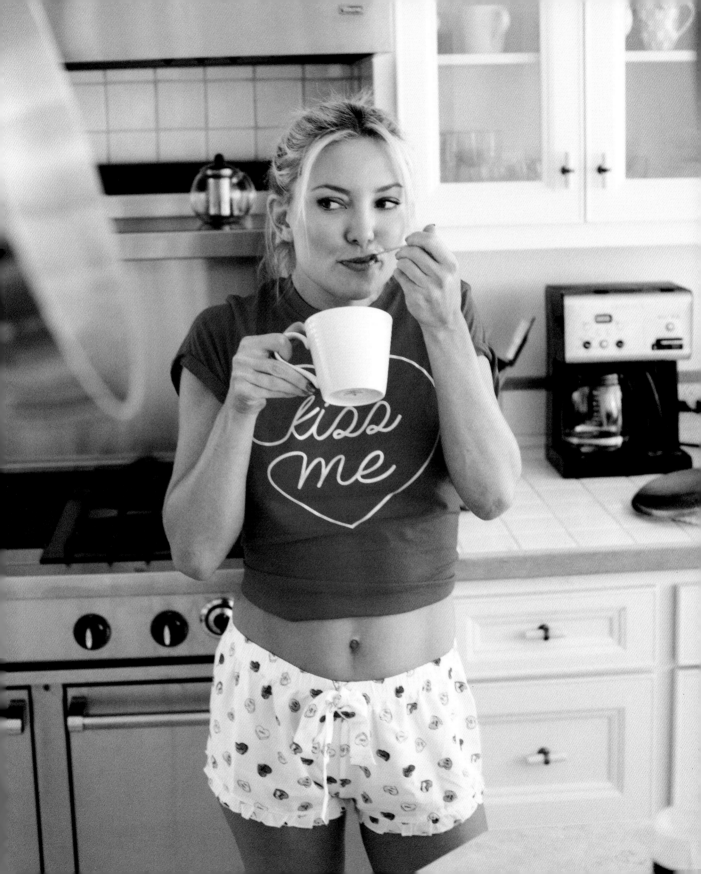

NOT-SO-GOOD FOOD LIST

HIGH IN SUGAR

Barbecue sauce

Cakes/cupcakes

Candy

Cocktail sauce

Condiments (ketchup, mayonnaise)

Cookies

Ice cream

Jams and jellies

Most nutrition bars

STARCHY CARBS WITH LITTLE FIBER

Cakes

Cookies

Doughnuts

Matzo

Packaged or instant oatmeal

Pastries

Pies

Pretzels

Rolls

Sweetened cereals

White or enriched pasta

White rice

DAIRY

Cream cheese

Cream or half-and-half

Frozen yogurt

Full-fat cheese

Ice cream

Milk

Sour cream

BAD FATS

All trans fats

Butter

Margarine

HIGHLY ACIDIC FOODS TO AVOID

Alcohol

Artificial sweeteners

Beef

Chicken*

Cocoa

Coffee and black tea

Dairy

Dried fruit

Eggs*

Full-fat cheese

Honey

Jam and jelly

Maple syrup

Mushrooms

Mustard

Pork*

Rice syrup

Shellfish

Soy sauce

Vinegar

*Indicates foods that have a highly acidic effect on the body; for more on the harmful effects of highly acidic foods, see page 105.

ACIDIC VS. ALKALINE FOODS

Our bodies are one large chemistry experiment. One way that our bodies try to assert their internal intelligence is by keeping pH levels in check. pH is a measure of how acidic or alkaline something is. Our blood pH needs to maintain a slightly alkaline level to keep us healthy. The problem is that all processed foods, and even some whole foods, can cause a highly acidic impact when ingested. We help our bodies maintain inner harmony by eating more alkaline-forming foods and fewer acid-forming foods.

* Alkaline-forming foods include most fruits, vegetables, herbs, nuts, seeds, and herbal teas.
* Acid-forming foods include most grains, beans, meats, dairy products, fish, fast foods, and processed foods.

Why is this important? When we eat acid-forming foods, our body has to work hard to bring our blood pH back into balance. It does this by releasing alkaline-rich minerals such as calcium, phosphorus, and magnesium into our bloodstream.

If we are not eating enough alkaline-forming foods, our body has to pull these important minerals from our bones, teeth, and organs. This can compromise our immune system, cause fatigue, and make us vulnerable to viruses and diseases.

But like most things, eating more alkaline does not mean all or nothing. A good rule of thumb is to try to go for a diet of 60 to 80 percent alkaline-forming foods and 20 to 40 percent acid-forming foods. Check out the Good Food List (page 101) and see which foods have a high acid impact. You can also take a look at the complete Alkaline and Acidic Foods List on page 229.

Making Meals Can Be Easy

I UNDERSTAND IT'S HARD and time-consuming to always prepare food from scratch for every meal. However, eating fresh food instead of food out of a box is part of the effort that has to go into changing your lifestyle. What I do is cook in bulk one day a week. Yes, I do cook! By doing it this way, I have time set aside to shop and cook—usually on a Sunday—when I'm relaxed. I cook enough to feed me and my boys. As you put together your meals, remember the four rules for eating well. Use the Good Food List (page 101) as inspiration and try to bulk prep some of your meals ahead of time.

Here's how I bulk prep the healthy building blocks of a week's worth of meals:

1. I make a list of all my basic ingredients for the week and I head to the market or grocery store.
2. Upon returning home, I lay everything out and crank up some great tunes.
3. I get out my supplies: glass containers in a variety of sizes (try to avoid Tupperware or other plastic containers, which can leach chemicals into your foods—more on that in chapter 7), skillet or sauté pan, steamer, rice cooker, blender, and several large mixing bowls.
4. Then I prepare several dishes and meals. Opposite, I've listed some of my go-to favorite dishes and foods that I prepare in advance for the week. I build on top of these. For example, if I make a big batch of quinoa, beans, and lentils, then I can mix and match to create different meals—such as quinoa with avocado and other veggies one day and lentil tacos on another day. The point is to have already prepared those foods that take a while to cook.

Breakfast
* Oatmeal (rolled oats, steel-cut oats, buckwheat)
* Fresh eggs (you can make hard-boiled or soft-boiled ahead of time and keep them on hand in the fridge)
* Protein-rich pancakes/waffles
* Sliced avocados doused in lemon juice
* Sliced fruit in small containers to take with you when you run out the door

Lunch/Dinner
* Large tossed salads
* Baked kale chips
* Red wine or rice wine vinegar and olive oil, combined for ready-to-go salad dressing
* Brown/wild rice, quinoa, millet, and sweet potatoes
* Grilled chicken, tuna steaks, roasted turkey
* Lentils, chickpeas, black beans, navy beans, black-eyed peas, tempeh, organic tofu
* Homemade vegetable soup, chili, butternut squash soup, split pea soup, or chicken soup
* Hummus; guacamole; homemade salsa; fruit butters; cashew cheese; individual serving sizes of nut butters, like almond, cashew, or sunflower seed

Snacks
* Homemade trail mixes (raw, unsalted varieties of nuts/seeds; raisins and dried cranberries; shredded coconut, etc.)
* Snack-sized containers of fresh cut veggies and fresh fruit
* Snack-sized containers of granola or our favorite gluten-free crackers

When bulk prepping is happening in my kitchen, it is usually a pretty big mess—pots going, blenders whirring. But having big batches of my go-tos on hand, like brown rice, quinoa, soups, and lentils, makes eating right during the week so much easier. So turn up your favorite tunes, get out your chopping board, and give it a try.

As you prepare these foods, cook them as simply as possible using little or no oil. Whenever possible, try steaming or grilling your proteins instead of pan-frying. Instead of salt, sugar, or butter, use lots of herbs and spices for great flavor. When you're ready to eat, a quick warming up in a skillet or in a preheated oven in your glass containers makes prep as easy as can be.

Instead of salt, sugar, or butter, use lots of herbs and spices for great flavor.

IT'S EASY TO BULK PREP

* Makes eating at home easier because you always have something ready

* Saves you time from cooking throughout the week

* Keeps you on track with your weight loss and goal of eating well

* Great for the budget!

* Keeps you away from packaged meals and quick-grab convenience foods!

I also understand that many people don't live near grocery stores that offer a lot of fresh produce and that good fresh produce tends to be expensive. In such cases, I recommend seeking out larger superstores such as Costco and Target—both of which have increased their offerings of frozen organic fruits, vegetables, dairy, and lean meats.

When You're Out of Balance

I HOPE BY NOW you're getting a clearer, stronger sense of your body—its physical, mental, and emotional tendencies, when you feel good and in balance, and when you start to feel out of balance. For all of us, no matter our primary type (or dosha), when we start to feel fatigued and tired and worn out, that's a pretty clear signal that our bodies are out of balance. Here are some quick ways to restore balance, depending on your primary type.

* **Vata:** You want to counteract your tendency to be light by eating warm, heavy, oily, and sweet foods. Home-cooked stews and soups, gluten-free pasta dishes, and even some homemade bread with olive oil will begin to put you back in balance.

* **Pitta:** When Pittas are out of balance, they tend to ignite their inner fire a bit too much. Usually this hits the digestive system with stomach upset, diarrhea, or inflammation. Try to cool down your system with sweet, bitter, and astringent tastes, including salads, raw veggies, beans, and lentils. This is also a time when you should avoid meat and try to go more vegetarian, staying away from the spicy foods you tend to enjoy!

* **Kapha:** When Kaphas are out of balance, they feel not just slow but lethargic. You need to reduce foods that are sweet and salty and instead go for lighter foods such as salads and raw vegetables, and try some spicy dishes and stir-fries. Small amounts of caffeine might also help Kaphas wake up from their slumberous state.

If you are a mix of two types, then look at your symptoms. Go back and see which of your ailments point to which dosha, and make adjustments that way. Start simply by taking out processed foods, gluten, or sugar. Those three are the worst offenders and can make anyone feel out of balance! (For more on using a cleanse to reset your balance, see chapter 7.)

Eat All Six Tastes in a Day!

DO YOU KNOW we have six different tastes? We do! Sweet, sour, salty, bitter, pungent, and astringent. In Ayurveda, it's recommended to include all six tastes during a day's eating to not only keep your taste buds and digestive system stimulated but also to make sure you get complete nutrition. So think of this as another way you can stoke your body's energetic fire!

Here's a quick guide to enlivening your taste buds.

* **Sweet:** You may think that all sweets are in the form of sugary foods—not so. In Ayurveda, sweet is associated with meat, oils, butter, milk, some grains, and, of course, fruits.
* **Sour:** citrus fruits; fermented foods such as pickles; dairy such as yogurt, sour cream, and cheese; vinegar and alcohol.
* **Salty:** This one is pretty easy to recognize—any food with added salt!
* **Bitter:** Want to know why kids don't like leafy greens and other vegetables? Because they are bitter!
* **Pungent:** Pungent tastes are present in spices, hot peppers, garlic, onions, and ginger.
* **Astringent:** This is not quite a true taste, but these foods have a "drying" effect on the body and include lentils, beans, and green tea.

Your Drawing Board: Food Exercise

NOW IS A good time to go to your *Drawing Board* and free associate. Write down a list of all your favorite go-to foods. Don't hold back. Be honest.

Next, write down a list of all the foods you ate in the past twenty-four hours. Go hour by hour, starting with breakfast (or the first meal you ate). If you can, note the time and place you ate. The more detail you can recall, the better.

Go back over the two lists and circle those foods that are on the Good Food List (page 101) and underline all the foods that you think fall into the not-so-good category.

* ✶ Don't do anything else. Just sit with your lists and think about them.
* ✶ Do you think you can live without any of those items that are on your not-so-good list?
* ✶ Are there foods from the Good Food List that you are missing but might enjoy?
* ✶ What food can you add to your go-to foods this week?

Keep it simple. Don't try to change too much too fast. Do one food exchange at a time. And continue to refer to this list, change it, and add to it.

Eating Intuitively

A REMARKABLE THING HAPPENS when you eliminate the junk from your diet: the cravings for fatty, sugar-laden, and salty snacks will disappear. When you eat clean, whole foods regularly throughout the day and in proper portion sizes, your body will no longer have the highs and lows in energy that come with cravings. Then, when you do have one of these indulgent treats every once in a while, your body will have built up a resistance to the swings. Eating in this way establishes a constancy of blood sugar that translates into more calm and clarity so that you reinforce that intuitive understanding of your body's needs.

Eating well will soon become second nature to you. The more whole foods and the fewer processed sweet and salty foods you eat, the stronger your brain-body signals become. Your body will let you know if the way you're eating is good or bad for you. And if you've indulged in a little too much of something that is not so good every once in a while—no big deal. Simply go back to your Drawing Board, record what you ate and how it made you feel, and pick up where you left off!

CHAPTER FIVE

PILLAR THREE

AWAKEN YOUR BODY

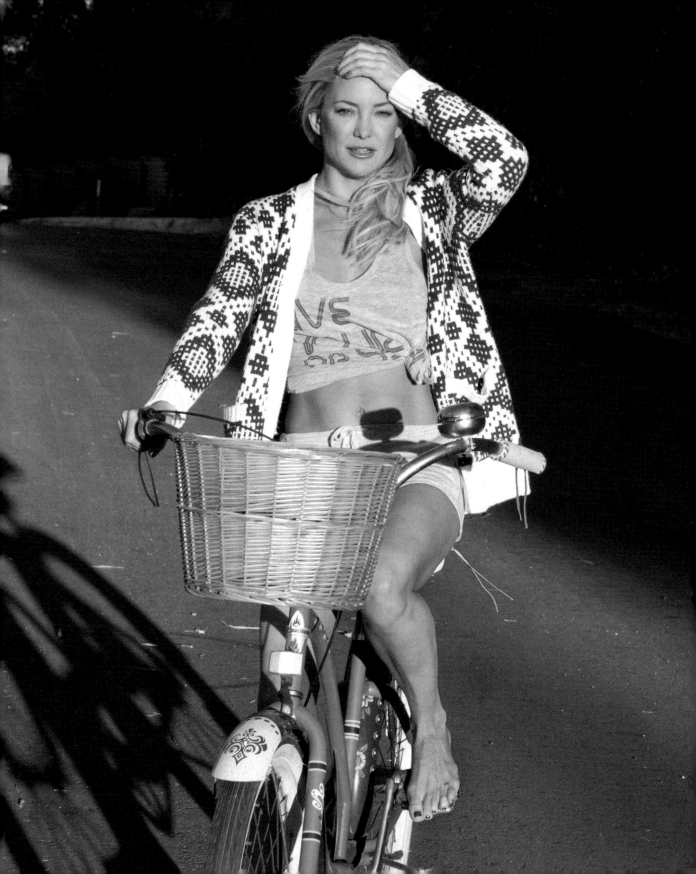

B Y NOW YOU must know that I'm in constant motion, I get bored easily, and I'm almost addicted to change. This is particularly true when it comes to how I work out. I wish I could say that I am still that kid who ran from soccer practice to dance lessons—only to fall asleep in a heap and get up and do it all again the next day!

When I wasn't dancing or playing soccer, I was outside on my bike or hiking around our ranch—especially when we lived in Colorado. Two of my brothers were older, so I was super motivated to keep up with them and their friends.

I still love to push my body—I love the exhilaration from a run, from working out hard, and from pushing myself to my limits. But that's me. You have your own unique relationship with your body and that's what this chapter is all about—fine-tuning your understanding of how you like to be and move in your body. The goal is to figure out what will make you *want* to exercise.

But all of us, regardless of our shape, size, weight, or interests, need to awaken our bodies from the inside out. We also need to understand our physical bodies, their shape and constitution, their average temperature and way of responding to certain types of environments, stimuli, and movement. Just like you learned in chapter 2, a strong starting place for making this connection is to figure out your general physical "type."

These categories are not black and white, and you might find yourself a bit of a hybrid—that's fine. The point is that you use this information as a way to begin thinking about how you want to get stronger, more fit, and toned—and lose weight, if that's your desire. This questionnaire is a continuation of the one you responded to in chapter 2. Record your answers in your Drawing Board and keep track of how your responses might begin to shift as you change your eating style and your activity level. You might also see subtle changes in your physical profile when you begin to integrate more mindfulness into your daily or weekly routine. But without a doubt, the more in touch you are with your body and its responses to stimuli around you, the more connected you will be to yourself. You will understand how you benefit from being more active and miss it when you skip it.

YOUR PHYSICAL PROFILE

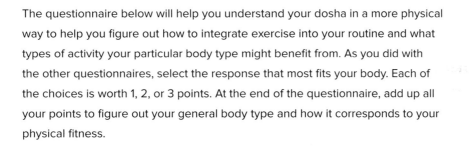

The questionnaire below will help you understand your dosha in a more physical way to help you figure out how to integrate exercise into your routine and what types of activity your particular body type might benefit from. As you did with the other questionnaires, select the response that most fits your body. Each of the choices is worth 1, 2, or 3 points. At the end of the questionnaire, add up all your points to figure out your general body type and how it corresponds to your physical fitness.

1. Amount of hair
   - ○ (1) Average
   - ○ (2) Thinning
   - ○ (3) Thick

2. Hair color
   - ○ (1) Light brown, blond
   - ○ (2) Red, auburn
   - ○ (3) Dark brown, black

3. Skin texture
   - ○ (1) Dry, rough, both
   - ○ (2) Soft, normal to oily
   - ○ (3) Oily, cool

4. Skin temperature
   - ○ (1) Cold hands, feet
   - ○ (2) Warm
   - ○ (3) Cold

5. Complexion
   - ○ (1) Dark
   - ○ (2) Pink, red
   - ○ (3) Pale, white

6. Eye size
   - ○ (1) Small
   - ○ (2) Medium
   - ○ (3) Large

7. Veins and tendons
- ◯ (1) Very prominent
- ◯ (2) Fairly prominent
- ◯ (3) Well covered

8. Whites of eyes
- ◯ (1) Blue/brown
- ◯ (2) Yellow/red
- ◯ (3) Glossy white

9. Teeth size
- ◯ (1) Very large or very small
- ◯ (2) Small to medium
- ◯ (3) Medium to large

10. Weight
- ◯ (1) Thin
- ◯ (2) Medium
- ◯ (3) Heavy, gains weight easily

11. Elimination
- ◯ (1) Dry, hard; often constipated
- ◯ (2) Soft to hard; frequent
- ◯ (3) Heavy, slow, thick; regular

12. Gender
- ◯ (1) Male
- ◯ (2) Female
- ◯ (3) Other

13. Heartbeats per minute
- ◯ (1) 70–90
- ◯ (2) 60–70
- ◯ (3) 50–60

14. Exercise tolerance
- ◯ (1) Low
- ◯ (2) Medium
- ◯ (3) High

15. Endurance
- ◯ (1) Fair
- ◯ (2) Good
- ◯ (3) Excellent

16. Strength
- ◯ (1) Fair
- ◯ (2) Better than average
- ◯ (3) Excellent

17. Speed
- ◯ (1) Very fast
- ◯ (2) Average
- ◯ (3) Not so fast

18. Competitiveness
- ◯ (1) Not at all competitive
- ◯ (2) Driven competitor/driven to win
- ◯ (3) Deal easily with competition

19. Walking speed

○ (1) Fast

○ (2) Average

○ (3) Slow and steady

20. Muscle tone

○ (1) Lean, low body fat

○ (2) Medium, good definition

○ (3) Large-bodied, bulky, high percentage of body fat

21. Animal you run like

○ (1) Deer

○ (2) Tiger

○ (3) Bear

22. Reaction time

○ (1) Quick

○ (2) Medium

○ (3) Slow

23. Body size

○ (1) Small frame, lean or long

○ (2) Medium frame

○ (3) Large frame, fleshy

WHAT YOUR RESPONSES MEAN

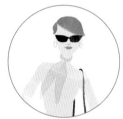

✳ **A score of 22 to 33 means that you are primarily Vata;** your dosha is composed of space and air. As a physical type, Vatas tend to be thin and lightning-quick on their feet—they move fast, walk fast, and even talk fast. They tend to be changeable and enthusiastic about new fads or fashions—their physical style is playful, resistant to routines, and sometimes forgetful of eating or sleeping enough, so they need to work on their strength and stability. Vatas like to swim, run, dance, and change it up! But they also lose interest quickly, so they need to challenge themselves to stick to a routine and be disciplined!

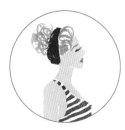

✳ **A score of 34 to 44 means that you are primarily Pitta,** which is symbolized by fire and water. Pitta types usually have medium builds, big eyes, and healthy glowing skin. Pittas like order and tend to be driven, competitive, and efficient. They don't like to waste time, so when they work out, they like the workout to be intense and to the point. They like challenges and learning new skills, sports, or activities. They like strategic sports such as mountain climbing, tennis, or archery. When in good health, Pittas will have strong constitutions, but when out of balance, they tend to have digestive issues. If Pittas don't stay in balance— through either food or physical or mental activity—they will feel out of sorts or become anxious and irritable. They can get too busy with work or other responsibilities and "forget" to work out, so the challenge for this dosha type is to make staying active a priority and remind yourself of how you benefit from exercise—mentally and physically.

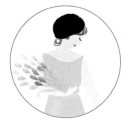

✳ **A score of 45 to 66 means that you are primarily Kapha.** Kaphas tend to be slow moving and thick bodied, with larger builds. They are big boned and can put on weight easily. They move slowly, talk and walk slowly, and don't really like to change their routines. In order to feel like they've had a good workout they need to sweat—this could be a slow but steady run or twenty minutes on an elliptical or rowing machine. When they are in balance, Kaphas are grounded and solid; when they are out of balance, they can overeat and develop excess mucus in the body, making them feel even more sluggish. The biggest challenge for Kaphas is a tendency to be lazy and lose motivation when they are out of balance. But since you are routine oriented, make your activity a habit and do it first thing in the morning!

Remember, all of us have some degree of each of the body types within us—we can also shift among the three depending on how active we are, what season it is, and the state of our overall health. To make this information useful and helpful, keep it in your Drawing Board. Check in with the questionnaire regularly to see how or if your responses are changing, and recognize any imbalance that might begin to emerge (see page 183 for more on how to check if your dosha is out of balance).

Awaken Your Body from the Inside

WHAT DO I mean by "awakening your body"? In short, it means breathing into your body and scanning it to connect with how it feels. Is your body tight? Restless? Achy? Relaxed? Weak? Strong?

* Do a quick body scan. Remember that exercise from chapter 2?
* Sit on a mat or in a chair.
* Breathe in through your nose and out through your mouth three times.
* Gently close your eyes.
* Scan your body from your head to your face, jaw, and neck.
* Go to your shoulders, upper back, between your shoulder blades.
* Scan your chest and abs and then move around to your lower back.
* Scan your torso, pelvis region, and your hips.
* Scan your arms and legs, your wrists and ankles.
* And finally, scan your feet.

How do you feel? Where is there discomfort? Tightness? Pain? Again, don't resist the sensation, but try instead to sit with it. Breathe into the area and then let go. Bring this body awareness to your day, especially if you have a source of discomfort that has just popped up.

Morning Stretch

I ALWAYS START OUT my day with an easy stretch and a body scan to see how I'm feeling—and sometimes I even begin this stretch while I'm still lying in bed! This slow movement is especially necessary when I'm working a lot, because I'm traveling and spending lots of time cooped up on a plane or in a car. This kind of focused attention on my body keeps me attuned and aware of the physical sensations. I feel a sense of peace. As you will see in chapter 6, I often pair this part of my morning routine with a quick mindfulness practice. The two together settle me, connect my body and mind, and make me feel calm and clear for the day ahead.

MY EASY MORNING STRETCH

✴ Starting position: Situate yourself on a soft mat or low-pile rug.

✴ Stand up (you can also sit in a straight-backed chair or do this stretch lying flat on your bed or the soft mat on the floor if either is more comfortable).

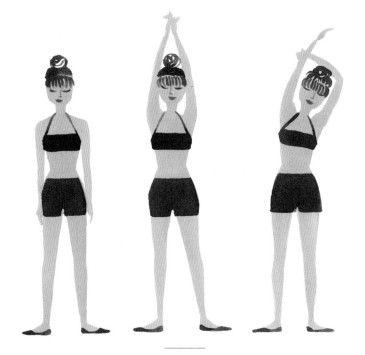

* Breathe in through your nose and out through your mouth.
* Stretch your arms over your head.
* Raise your left arm overhead, and, holding your left wrist, lean to your right side.
* Raise your arm overhead, and, holding your right wrist, lean to the left side.

LEG WARM-UP

* In an open squat position, bend into your thighs (3x).
* Lie down on your mat with your arms stretched above your head.

LEG STRETCHES

* Place a yoga strap, belt, or scarf around one foot. Keep your other leg bent at the knee and your foot on the mat. Gently stretch the straightened leg toward you (with a slight bend in your knee—don't lock it).
* Let the straight leg fall to one side, stretching the inner thigh.
* Then let it fall to the other side, stretching your calf and IT band.
* Reverse legs.

ROLLER

* Open up your chest and arms.
* Lay on a foam roller with it perpendicular to your body.
* Roll up and down your spine.
* Roll from your tail bone to the base of your head.
* Place your arms in "goal post" position, and move them up over your head and back down. Keep your arms on one plane, level to your body and with your shoulders down.

GENTLE SPINE TWISTS

✳ Lying flat on your back, bring one knee across your body.

✳ Stretch your arms out to either side.

✳ Try to keep your shoulders flat on the mat.

After this morning stretching routine, I feel energized and open, ready to start my day.

What Works for Me

MY APPROACH TO how I exercise is based on combining three forms of movement: cardio, strengthening, and toning or lengthening my muscles. I wish I could work out every day, but I don't. I try for four days a week, but some weeks it's only three days—I just don't have the time. But the reason this minimal approach works for me is that I figured out how to push my body just enough, change up the actual exercises so my body doesn't plateau, and alternate the types of exercise to maximize their effect. I know that probably sounds like a giant cliché, but I do think if you pay attention to what your body needs in three ways—aerobic fitness (through cardio exercises), strengthening (through weighted exercises), and toning (through stretching/sculpting/lengthening of the muscles)—you, too, can figure out some shortcuts to the body that you want, with minimal time commitment.

Ideally, what you're aiming for in any given week is this:

1. Work out four or five days a week for 30 to 60 minutes.
2. Alternate cardio, strength, and stretch/tone/sculpt (this means alternating within one workout or over consecutive days).

Realistically, what will keep you in shape is this:

1. Once or twice a week, go for a long, strenuous workout that includes 20 to 30 minutes cardio, 20 to 30 minutes strengthening, and 20 to 30 minutes stretch/tone/sculpt.
2. On two other days, do 15 minutes of either cardio, strength, or stretch/tone/sculpt.

One more thing: We all have different bodies and we all, more or less, have different ways we want to look. I like being slim and toned, yet strong. Since I'm athletic and can build muscle easily, if I do too much strength training, I start to add bulky muscle, which doesn't suit me. On the other hand, you might really like that look. It's up to you how you want to shape your own body.

Because it feels like I don't have enough time, I've become efficient at putting together some go-to routines—just like I do with my meal prep. Some days, I go to a Spin class—an intense 45- to 60-minute cardio workout to music. Other days, I go to a dance studio and do 2 to 3 hours of advanced jazz-modern, which hits all three of my goals—cardio, strengthening, and toning. And one of my all-time favorite workout classes is pole dancing. This is an intense, full-body workout that is so fun and fabulous—I recommend it to anyone with the guts to try it! Grab a friend or two and do it together—trust me, you'll laugh, move, and connect with that inner sexy diva who's dying to come out of her shell!

But my go-to workouts are at home, where I use music to work out to my own routines, or watch DVDs of 20- to 30-minute routines, including Pilates (toning), Insanity (strengthening), Brazilian Butt Lift (obvious!), and others. There are thousands of cool, fast workouts that you can watch and follow at home. And every day, more and more are available through online streaming. Check out Mary Helen Bowers's *Ballet Beautiful*—she has an awesome series for arms, legs, and core, all that lengthen, tone, and strengthen in the ways that professional ballet dancers train.

Twice a week, I try to do a *long* workout; a typical one includes:

- ✳ 30 minutes of dance cardio
- ✳ 30 minutes of butt and core
- ✳ 10 minutes of arm exercises (which typically means arm "shapeners" using low weights—I love Tracy Anderson's Method)
- ✳ A few short workouts (20 to 30 minutes) I do to a song or two:
  - First half of the song, I do tricep push-ups on my knees (resting in child's pose when I need to)
  - Second half of song, I do wide arm push-ups on my knees

Exercise really comes down to moving in a way that makes you feel good. I love music and dancing—that's my thing. You might love a short run or a walk around the block chatting with your girlfriends. Whatever works for you is what's best. But remember two really important points: 1) food is more important than you think; the more clean you eat, the more effective even short workouts will be; and 2) you absolutely need to switch up what you do for exercise so you don't get bored. Trust me on that one.

Go Outside!

I'M A NATURE girl! I never feel more alive and in harmony with myself as I do when I am outside, enjoying the beautiful outdoors. I can get lazy and sometimes have to push myself outside to remind myself how good it feels. My mind simply feels more space and peace and my body feels invigorated in fresh air. So this lesson is all about getting outside to awaken your body and strengthen its spirit. Try this quick exercise.

Imagine you are stepping lightly over grass and fallen leaves, your feet sinking into the softness. You hear a light crunch underneath as your feet, then legs, and then your arms begin to move and find

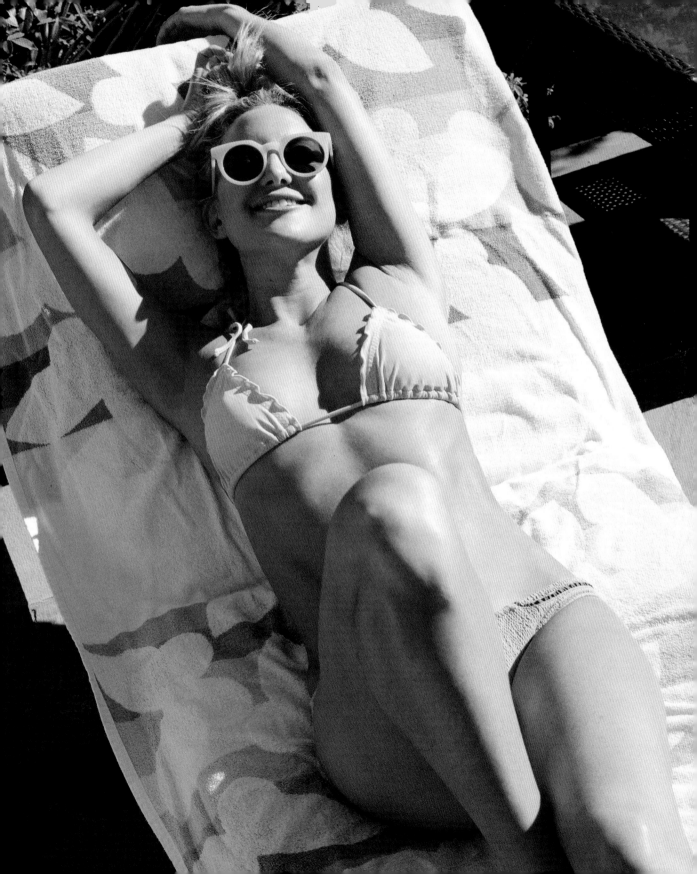

their rhythm. You notice the grass and leaves are still a bit wet from the dew—or did it rain last night? You don't mind. You breathe, taking in the slightly musty smell of the autumn leaves. You listen as birds call to one another. You hear cars passing in the distance. You let thoughts of the coming day pass through your mind, then you let them go into the ether. You breathe in, you breathe out. Your skin begins to tingle, and then you break a light sweat as your pace increases.

All your senses are alive as you feel the sun break through the tall trees, finding your face, warming it. You are moving through the morning air. You don't want to run—just walk more briskly. You begin to pump your arms, holding your elbows in tightly to increase your pace. Feeling through your feet, the ground seems to be talking to you. You feel the muscles down the entire length of your legs flex and release as you move. Your abs are firm, your back feels strong and supple, and the tightness in your hips and aches in your knees have become memories. You breathe in and out. It's the start of a new day, a new day to move your body, awaken your mind, and renew and revitalize your spirit. Your body, mind, and heart thank you for this surge of adrenaline, endorphins, and energy. You've never felt clearer, stronger, and more comfortable in your own skin.

This is not just a fantasy. This could be you, when you step outside and use the natural environment as your workout space. From mountain trails to suburban parks, from hillsides to beaches, from nearby woods to city streets. The world is waiting for you to explore.

Being outside will not only connect us to the power of nature but also to ourselves. When we are outside, we are activated—our minds, brains, and our bodies. We breathe in more oxygen and our bodies relax—even when we are moving. Also, it's hard to stay sedentary for long when you're outdoors. You have to move—even if it's a lazy walk down the street.

———

But the really amazing experience that we have when we are outside in the fresh air is what is called the biophilia effect (*biophilia* literally means "love of life"). Hypothesized by Harvard biologist E. O. Wilson in his 1984 book by the same name, biophilia is based on the idea that all living beings have an "innate affiliation to other living organisms."

I never knew that term until recently, but I've felt the truth of it in my bones since I was a little girl. Why is it so important for us to connect with nature and be outdoors? Because mounting research shows the profound effect that fresh air, plants, trees, and natural outdoor elements have on our health and well-being. When we spend time outdoors, especially while being active, we can literally shift our mood, become more positive in our thoughts, and feel more in harmony with ourselves and the world around us. Many of us know that we need sunlight in order to feel healthy and optimistic, and those who suffer from seasonal affective disorder (SAD) in the dark months of winter know this to be true even more intensely. This is the same principle, taken a step further: As human beings we need not only natural sunlight but to stay connected to nature in order to feel our best, do our best, and be our best. And though recent studies have shown that being in a natural, outdoor environment is one of the very best things you can do for your health, amazingly, working Americans typically spend 92 percent of each day indoors. Tina Vindum, former Olympic downhill racer, outdoor fitness trainer, and author, has done a ton of research on the benefits of exercise in the outdoors; here's what she says you are missing out on:

＊ Levels of serotonin, a neurotransmitter that helps regulate our mood, rise when we are outside. A study at the University of Queensland found that regular outdoor runners were less anxious and depressed than people who ran indoors on a treadmill, and had higher levels of post-exercise endorphins (the feel-good brain chemicals associated with runner's high).

* Exposure to nature reduces pain and illness and speeds recovery time. In one study of postoperative patients, those who had rooms with a view of natural surroundings needed less pain medication and spent fewer days in the hospital than those who faced a brick wall. In another study among prisoners in Michigan, those who were able to view sky, grass, and trees had 24 percent fewer infirmary visits and significantly fewer digestive illnesses and headaches.

* Being in nature reduces stress-related anger and enhances sociability. Frances Kuo, a researcher at the University of Illinois, has shown that being around grass and greenery reduces rates of domestic violence and school truancy and leads to better grades and increased social interaction. And a study by Dr. David Lewis, the man who coined the term *road rage,* found that the scent of grass has a significant calming effect on out-of-control drivers.

* You also do your lungs a favor when you exercise outdoors: According to the Environmental Protection Agency, indoor air in the United States is two to five times more polluted than outdoor air (meaning outdoor air is 75 percent less polluted than indoor air!). Fresh air is also rich in negative ions (oxygen molecules with an extra electron). These negative ions have been linked to improved sense of well-being, heightened awareness and alertness, decreased anxiety, and a lower resting heart rate.

I love all these fun facts! And what's better than spending time outdoors? Exercising outdoors! It's simply a biological fact that our bodies are programmed to find the easiest way to complete tasks they possibly can. So in a gym workout, whether using cardio equipment, free weights, or a circuit training machine, your body will quickly learn what it has to do, which is why people reach a plateau so quickly and why the results produced in a gym setting eventually lessen. But in the outdoors, your body is constantly adapting as it moves up, down, diagonally, or side to side. Outdoors you aren't doing the same thing over and over again. Think of taking a walk down a hill or even on a sidewalk. You have to make slight adjustments to rocks on the path or cracks in the sidewalk. That is information that stimulates your brain and body to make certain adjustments. Not only does this keep your body and brain active and engaged but you are continually challenging yourself, becoming stronger, faster, and smarter.

Being outside also appeals to our sense of play and adventure. Like I've said, I spent my childhood outside! And most of us do—we run, jump and skip. Why not reactivate this sense of play and fun for ourselves now?!

EXERCISE AND YOUR BRAIN

The research is in. The conclusions are drawn. Exercise stimulates the brain's ability to focus and concentrate, strengthens our ability to learn and remember, and helps us create more brain cells and connections. In a powerful, consistent way, every time we exercise, increase our heart rate, and pump oxygen through our blood, we are giving our brains fuel to generate new neurons. This is called neurogenesis and it's at the root of why our brains are plastic (able to change, adapt, and grow). So if you thought exercise was good for just your body, think again. Exercise can actually make you smarter! Check out the work of Dr. Wendy Suzuki, a neuroscientist from New York University who has done amazing studies that show this connection between exercise and the brain! In several experiments using herself and her undergraduate students as subjects, she has shown how our long-term memory improves through short-term exercise; her studies have also pointed to how those feel-good endorphins are just the tip of the iceberg. Exercise, especially any form that is aerobic and gets your heart pumping, creates new neurons—talk about smart!

Your Drawing Board: Movement

GET OUT YOUR *Drawing Board*. You need to ask yourself some questions about how you move throughout the day. Remember, be honest. This is just a record of where you are right now, not where you'll be forever.

* What is your current morning routine to awaken your body?
* How do you like to stretch?
* Are you feeling Vata, Pitta, or Kapha today?
* How often do you spend time outside?
* When you are outside, what do you do?
* Have you ever exercised before work? Do you feel more energized and focused when you do?
* Do you have any physical limitations that get in the way of exercising regularly?
* How often do you exercise each week, including taking a short walk?
* When you walk upstairs, do you ever get short of breath?
* Do you have trouble going up or down stairs?
* Can you balance on one leg?

Your responses to these questions should give you a basic sense of your overall physical condition. If you're exercising regularly, you most likely will not be short of breath going up stairs. If you do have some physical limitations (a knee or hip injury, for instance), you might be inhibited from walking or doing other forms of exercise. If you are frequently spending time outside, then you are most likely fairly active—walking, running, biking, gardening, or playing sports. However, spending less than one hour per week outdoors might point to a sedentary lifestyle.

Regardless of your responses, be honest but gentle with yourself. This is neither a contest nor an indictment. It's a place to begin.

Choosing What to Do

I AM NOT IN a position to tell you what to do when it comes to diet, exercise, or anything else. I can share only the information that I've learned about how important exercise is to our bodies, brains, and minds. It's really up to you to make a commitment to integrate exercise into your daily routine. Try to do some kind of physical check-in with yourself every day. That doesn't have to mean exercising by running or working out. It could mean that you just do a body scan, or awaken your body with a stretch. Maybe you just take a walk around the block or the office parking lot. The point is to connect with your body in a physical way.

But . . .

If you do really want to get in better shape, lose weight, wear those jeans or yoga pants with more confidence, then start by figuring out how and what you can do. I've created the seven Movement Profiles on pages 134–135 to capture a wide range of activities and ways to get exercise. Here's the challenge:

For one week, choose one activity in one category and commit to doing it three times. That's it. One activity, three times in one week.

SIGN YOUR NAME HERE:

_____

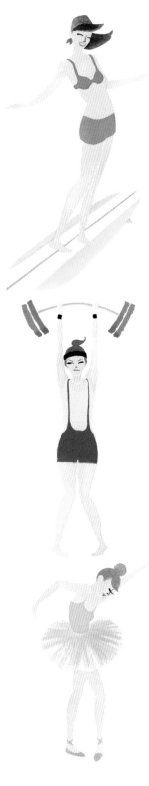

Be an Explorer
(yoga, surfing, paddle-boarding, climbing)

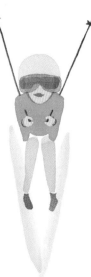

Be a Mover
(running, walking, cycling, Spinning, skiing)

Be a Strengthener
(weight lifting, CrossFit, gym exercises)

Be a Dancer
(Zumba, ballroom dancing, and everything in between)

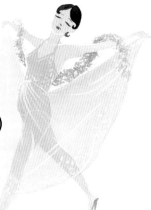

Be a Toner
(Pilates, barre, ballet-based class, core classes, sculpt classes)

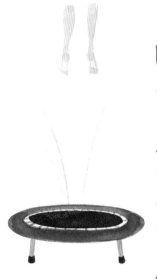

Be a Player

(meaning be playful—hula hooping, jumping rope, AcroJam, trampoline jumping, dodgeball, kick the can, KanJam, Ultimate Frisbee, playing with your kids)

Be a Competitor

(swimming, tennis, squash, basketball, volleyball)

After giving lots of different types of activities a try, you will quickly identify the kind of movement you like best. And when you identify your "type," it might be easier for you to commit to a routine! Keep in mind, you don't have to be one type—as you know, I change it up all the time!

Remember, exercise has many benefits. It:

* Reduces stress
* Improves attention and memory
* Restores mental energy and stamina
* Increases longevity
* Strengthens our bones, heart, skin

Staying active pumps energy into our body and our brains and makes us feel alive!

DRAWING BOARD

Imagine yourself at nine years old. What did you do? What activities did you enjoy? Imagine yourself doing those activities. Might you be able to do them again?

THE INNER CALM OF A SUN SALUTATION

Some days when I'm feeling kind of quiet and slow, I awaken my body with a Sun Salutation, a twelve-pose (asana) series that opens my mind, body, and spirit. This series of poses puts me in sync with my breath, helps me connect to my body, and gets my blood moving just enough.

1. Salutation (inhale, exhale), hands in Namaste
2. Raise arms, inhale
3. Extend into forward bend, exhale
4. Forward lunge, right leg, inhale
5. (Stand up, exhale)
6. Downward-Facing Dog, inhale
7. (Stand up, exhale)
8. Eight limbs
9. Cobra
10. (Stand up)
11. Downward-Facing Dog
12. Forward lunge, left leg, inhale
13. (Stand up, exhale)
14. Forward bend
15. Raise arms overhead
16. Salutation, exhale

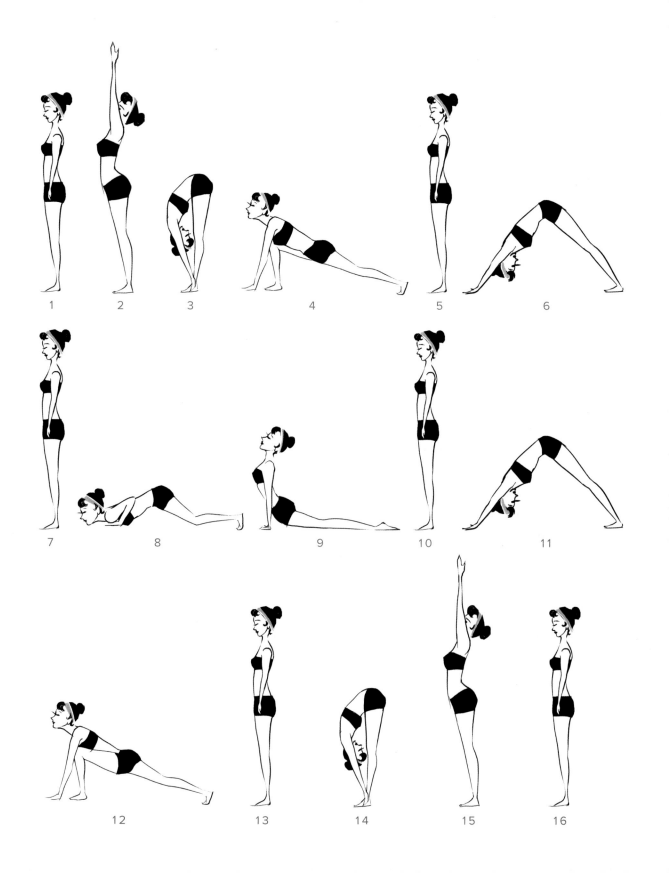

1   2   3   4   5   6

7   8   9   10   11

12   13   14   15   16

Change Is My Constant

AS YOU CAN probably tell by now, I like to try new things—new foods, new exercises, new beauty routines, new ways to wear my hair. In fact, that's probably the biggest constant in my life—change. I change my routine. I change my look. I change my mind. Some of this need to change is so I don't get bored—heaven forbid. But some of this desire for novelty comes from a built-in need to adapt and keep my mind and body sharp.

I've asked myself: Is this a blessing or a curse? Am I so changeable that I don't stick with things? Or is my need for change just an extension of my adventurous spirit? Probably both. But here's the thing: I thrive on change. Here's another thing: I don't care anymore what it means. I don't seek to judge myself and I don't want to get caught in the quicksand of self-analysis. I'm just me and I've accepted myself—warts and all.

When it comes to exercise and making sure I bring it into every day, I remind myself of all that I like and enjoy.

When it comes to exercise and making sure I bring it into every day, I remind myself of all that I like and enjoy. I use my Drawing Board to remind myself of what I like to do, and I do it!

Your Drawing Board

I just ate: Spaghetti

WHAT DO YOU like to do? What new activity do you want to try? What is something that scares you but you want to find the courage to give it a whirl? Get out your *Drawing Board* and make a list!

Once you make your list, identify the type of exercise: Is it cardio? A strengthener? A toner? Sometimes exercises—like interval training—combine all three. The more you are aware of how an exercise affects your body, the more flexible you will be putting your own routines together.

But the most important part is to get used to moving. Start simply—with a daily walk. Add in a stretch so that you become more aware of how tight or open you are in your joints and muscles. The more you begin to move, the more your body will signal to you—and more than likely it will tell you, "This feels great!"

CHAPTER SIX

PILLAR FOUR

THE MIRACLE OF MINDFULNESS

EDITATION HAS SAVED my sanity. Not that I was crazy, but in this world of hyperspeed, overstimulation, no escape from technology, and constant emotional stress, it's very hard to stay centered and grounded. And yet, since I've integrated meditation into my daily life—which doesn't mean I do it every day—I feel so much more at ease, knowing that I can re-center myself when life feels out of control.

I first learned the importance of a mindfulness practice from my mom. In so many ways she was an amazing role model. Although she began meditating a long time ago, and I observed it as part of her regular routine, over the past few years she has taken up a cause to teach the world about how mindfulness practice can help children strengthen their emotional intelligence. So it has been from her that I first learned about the vast and amazing neuroscience research that shows the many cognitive, emotional, physical, and spiritual benefits that come from integrating a mindfulness practice into our lives.

During one particularly difficult time in my life when I was feeling overwhelmed, it was meditation that brought me back to me. At the time, a tough decision left me feeling completely upended. I could not stop my mind from racing. I could barely sleep. And I felt trapped by my anxiety. My mom told me to just start simply, by calming down and bringing awareness to my breaths. She told me to follow my breaths in and out, remembering that the thoughts would come, but to just watch them pass, and to always come back to a simple breath.

At first, I felt even more uncomfortable in my body and mind when I tried this. I felt like squirming away, like a toddler in time-out. But I kept at it, trusting my mom when she said it would get easier, and that you got more comfortable.

And soon, I felt it starting to work. I practice meditation regularly now, sometimes even twice a day—in the morning and again before I go to bed.

It's not always easy, but afterward I always feel relief. I sigh, I exhale. Meditation varies just like everything else. Sometimes it feels like I can sit for hours. Other times, I feel like that toddler again, squirming out of my seat. On other, special days, I arrive at amazing insights and experience a huge release of emotions I didn't even know were bottled in.

I think often people turn to meditation when they are having difficult times like I did, but it doesn't require bad times to get started. And I realize that mindfulness is all the rage these days, but I have to urge you to consider this as a really important pillar to your overall wellness and self-care plan. Still not convinced? Okay, let's take a step back and see how stressed you are.

The Antidote to Stress

WHY HAS MINDFULNESS become so popular? Why are so many scientists—from neuroscientists to physicists to physicians and psychologists and biologists—jumping on the so-called bandwagon of meditation? Because all of us are feeling so stressed! And meditation and mindfulness practices have been shown to relieve stress. Doing ten to fifteen minutes of meditation (or any other form of mindfulness practice) lowers blood pressure, calms the nervous system, and boosts the immune system.

For me, I've never felt healthier or more calm, clear, and content in my life as I have since making mindfulness part of my daily routine. This does not mean I sit down cross-legged on the floor and chant for an hour. It doesn't mean I go to a meditation class every morning or evening—though both of those options exist for those who are inclined. Mindfulness for me comes down to four simple things:

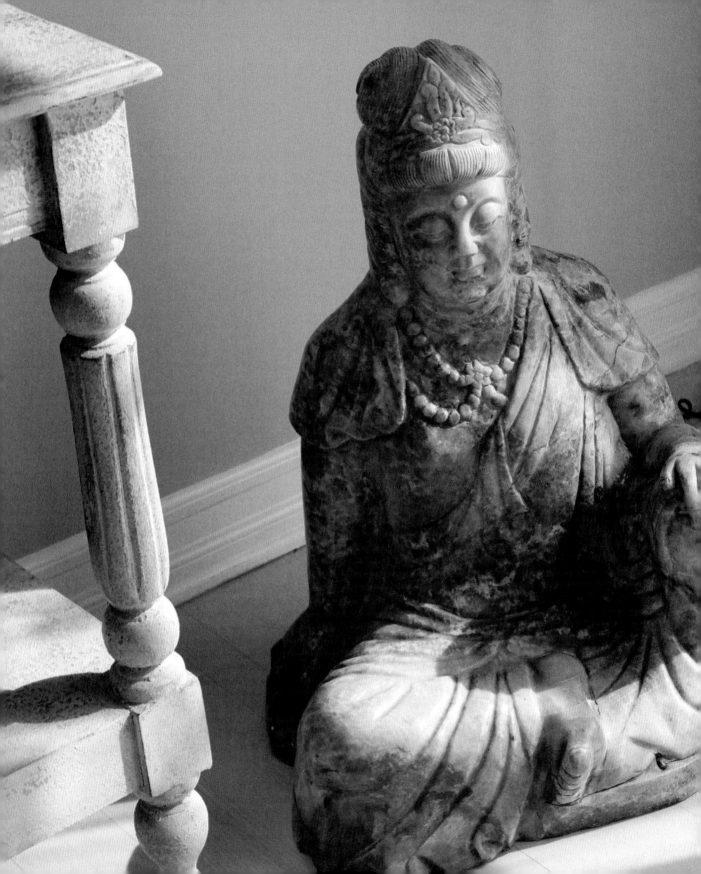

Let your teacher
be love itself.
— Rumi

———

* Connecting with my breath in a conscious way
* Using this conscious breathing to become aware of my thoughts and feelings
* Actively observing my thoughts and feelings
* Letting go of these thoughts and feelings and letting my mind simply wander

Sometimes I do sit on a soft mat and go through a guided meditation (listening to an audio recording of a guide cueing me to certain steps). Sometimes I go through a few yoga poses while I meditate, connecting with my breath and body as a way to settle myself and then laying in *shavasana* (corpse pose). And sometimes I go for a walk in nature and do what I call a "walking meditation," in which I walk while listening on my phone to a soothing instrumental song or music of the sea shore, a babbling brook, or some other melodic piece. I let the rhythm of the music sync with my gait.

For me, sometimes meditating is simply stopping what I am doing, sitting down cross-legged, closing my eyes, and breathing in through my nose and out through my mouth for five minutes. I often do this during a hectic workday.

Other times, my meditation is just staring at a wall. I don't try to do anything—I am just being quiet with myself, letting my thoughts wander.

You can meditate or practice mindful awareness in thousands of different ways—one is no better or more valuable than another. It's all about the intention you put toward it and what works for you.

Notice I did not use the word *effort*. Mindfulness is the exact opposite of putting forth effort. Mindfulness is part relaxation and part focus. In fact, scientists actually distinguish between two basic types of meditation approaches that are related and support each other:

1. Focused attention
2. Open monitoring

———

Focused attention is an approach that trains your mind to keep your flow of attention on one certain object or idea—a chant or mantra, a prayer, counting your breaths. The idea is that when we train our minds to maintain focus on one thing, we let go of all the other random thoughts that distract us—our worries, our thoughts of the future, our to-do lists. When we focus on one stream of thought, we strengthen our resistance to distraction.

Open monitoring is almost the opposite of focused attention. It's when you learn to observe your thoughts and feelings without attachment or judgment. Think of it this way: You are lying down in the middle of an open field on a bright summer day. You are relaxed and at ease. You don't have a care in the world. You feel safe and content. Above you the sky is filled with passing clouds. Your only activity is to watch the clouds pass. You take note of their shape, their color. But that's it.

Open monitoring is similar to that experience of watching the clouds go by: You're watching, paying attention, but you don't get stuck on any one thought. You watch, have thoughts, and feelings go by without judgment, without attachment, without tension. You stay open to whatever might occur in the mind or body. You notice sights, sounds, smells, and feelings—but without responding. When you practice this kind of meditative exercise, you are aware but nonreactive.

Many new and popular guided meditation practices offer a combination of these two approaches. For instance, someone will lead you to focus on your breath, maybe even count your breaths, to settle your mind and train your focus on one thing. Then, after a few minutes, the guide will suggest that you just let your mind wander, to resist focus and control.

But no matter what the meditation or mindfulness practices, each has the same goal, just different paths: calmness, clarity, and contentment. All mindfulness practices can help us to find a balance of focus and relaxation—in both mind and body. And this is why it's so powerful. It helps us create more mental energy for what really matters.

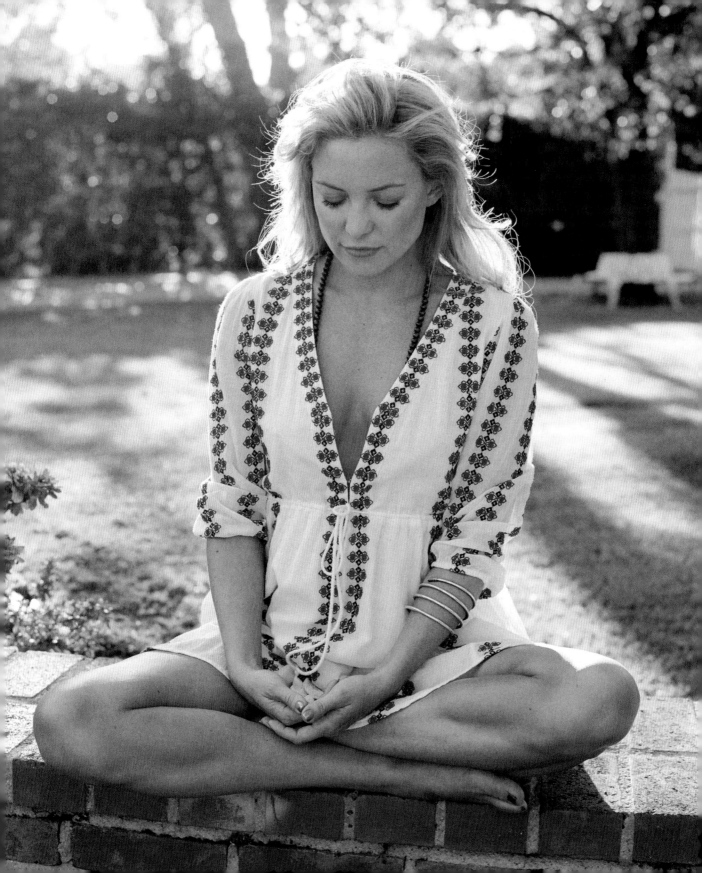

STRESS CAN BE GOOD!

We all know that too much stress is bad for us, and that's true. But having some stress is actually good—it keeps us on our toes and builds our emotional endurance. A moderate amount of stress activates our brains and bodies, enabling us to have sharper focus. So the next time you feel stressed, try to reframe it: "Hey, self—this stress is good!"

It's a reframe.

In the past, any time I felt mounting stress in my life, I crawled into bed and cried. Now I say to myself, "Okay, this doesn't feel good, but I can get through it." And it works.

Don't underestimate the power of saying things out loud!

So How Stressed Are You?

STRESS IS NOT only in your head. When we experience stress, it directly affects our bodies and our brains. Although we are biologically designed to deal with stress (a hardwired reaction to either flee from trouble or danger or stand up and fight), our brains have not really caught up with how to manage modern-day stress. In other words, from an evolutionary point of view, our stress response was designed to protect us from predators—tigers and lions on the savannah. But today, our brains respond to all sorts of stimuli as stressful—criticism from a boss, too much work without sufficient downtime, worry over children or parent health. The source of stress matters less than how we perceive these triggers for stress. Unfortunately, our brains still go through the same cycle they always have—releasing cortisol, a hormone that floods our brains and causes that uptight, worried, anxious feeling. Too much cortisol literally wears down our hearts (creates the spike in blood pressure and link to heart attacks and heart disease), our immune systems, and our ability to think clearly. Together, all of these negative stress responses take away our ability to experience contentment and joy. They lead to depression and anxiety. They rob us of our well-being. So now that you know how destructive stress can be, let's see how stressed you are. Respond to the questions below and form a baseline of your day-to-day stress.

STRESS QUESTIONNAIRE

This questionnaire will help you determine both how stressed you are on a daily basis and how you tend to manage that stress. Stress is inevitable and ubiquitous. There truly is no escape. But we can change our orientation to it and learn more productive, effective coping mechanisms. To that end, respond to the following questions and choose the response that best fits you most of the time.

1. Do you find yourself eating emotionally as a response to stress or difficult feelings (eating unhealthy foods or eating when you're not hungry)?

○ (3) No, I eat a healthy diet and only eat when I'm hungry.

○ (2) I admit I've binged on the occasional Häagen Dazs, but it's not a regular occurrence.

○ (1) Yes, I have to admit that my diet is generally unhealthy.

2. Do you find yourself sweating excessively when you're not exercising?

○ (3) No.

○ (2) Sometimes, when I'm particularly stressed, but not often.

○ (1) Yes, it happens fairly regularly.

3. Do you ever have trouble sleeping?

○ (3) Rarely or never.

○ (2) Sometimes I'll have trouble falling asleep, staying asleep, or getting quality sleep.

○ (1) Yes, I often have trouble with sleep quality or with falling and staying asleep.

4. Are you experiencing any digestive problems, such as indigestion, IBS, constipation, or diarrhea?

○ (3) No.

○ (2) I get the occasional stress-related stomachache, but nothing too regular.

○ (1) Yes, I experience regular digestive problems.

5. Are you suffering from burnout, anxiety, or depression?

○ (3) No.

○ (2) I don't know.

○ (1) Yes.

6. Are you taking care of yourself?

○ (3) Yes, I take good care of my body and soul.

○ (2) I don't have as much time for self-care as I'd like, but I'm doing okay.

○ (1) No, I rarely take care of myself.

7. Do you have a supportive social network and take time for relationships in your life?

○ (3) Yes. My friends and family help a lot with stress.

○ (2) Somewhat. I have a few close relationships and can talk to people if something's really bothering me but don't have as much time for relationships as I'd like.

○ (1) No, I have few close friends or supportive family ties, or I don't have time to devote to the people I could be close with.

8. Are you getting regular exercise?

○ (3) Yes. I lead an active lifestyle and exercise at least three times per week.

○ (2) Sort of. I get some exercise throughout the day or I go to the gym a couple times a week.

○ (1) No. I live a sedentary lifestyle and don't go to the gym regularly.

9. Do you find yourself smoking and/or drinking to excess as a way to deal with stress?

○ (3) No.

○ (2) I do one of those things, but it's not a big problem for me.

○ (1) Yes, and to be honest, I know it can't be good for me.

10. Do you often experience headaches?

○ (3) No. I've had them before but not often.

○ (2) Sort of. I get them once a month or so.

○ (1) Yes, I struggle with them regularly.

11. Are you having trouble maintaining a healthy weight? Or are you carrying excessive abdominal fat?

○ (3) No, I'm within ten pounds of my "ideal" weight.

○ (2) To a degree. I struggle with my diet like many people, but it's not too much of a problem.

○ (1) Yes, I've put on much more weight than I'm comfortable with. / I can't keep weight off. / My problem area is my abdomen.

12. Are you easily irritated?

○ (3) No, I'm pretty even tempered. It takes quite a bit to get me flustered.

○ (2) Somewhat. I find I have less patience than I'd like, but it's not a problem in my life.

○ (1) Yes. I find myself snapping at people out of frustration, or having a low threshold for dealing with annoyances.

13. How often have you missed work in the past year due to illness?

○ (3) Maybe once.

○ (2) Two to three times.

○ (1) Four times or more.

14. Do you often feel fatigued at the end of a day?

○ (3) Not too much. I'm ready for sleep at night, but I do have energy in the evenings.

○ (2) Somewhat. I come home and need to rest for a while before I can do activities in the evenings.

○ (1) Yes. In fact, I'm often fatigued by the *middle* of the day.

15. Do you have a feeling that stress may be affecting your health?

○ (3) Not really. I'm just taking this test for fun.

○ (2) Possibly. I'm not sure, but I wouldn't be shocked if it were true.

○ (1) Yes. In fact, I'd be surprised if stress *weren't* affecting my health.

WHAT YOUR RESPONSES MEAN

In general, the lower your score, the more effectively you are managing the stress in your life. The higher your score, the more help you need to reconsider how you can more effectively manage your stress.

✳ If you scored a 15, you are doing a great job managing your stress. You have developed good coping mechanisms—good for you!

✳ If you scored between 16 and 30, you are experiencing moderate stress in your life but you seem to be able to manage it through physical activity, some mindfulness practice, and other ways of coping. You might want to think about how to increase some of these stress-reducing activities.

✳ If you scored between 31 and 45, you are experiencing a high amount of stress and it has begun to take a toll on your health. You would benefit from integrating some helpful stress-management tools, including meditation, physical exercise, relaxation breathing, journaling—and, of course, eating well and getting enough rest.

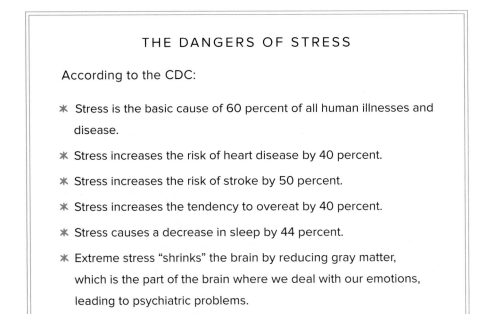

THE DANGERS OF STRESS

According to the CDC:

✳ Stress is the basic cause of 60 percent of all human illnesses and disease.

✳ Stress increases the risk of heart disease by 40 percent.

✳ Stress increases the risk of stroke by 50 percent.

✳ Stress increases the tendency to overeat by 40 percent.

✳ Stress causes a decrease in sleep by 44 percent.

✳ Extreme stress "shrinks" the brain by reducing gray matter, which is the part of the brain where we deal with our emotions, leading to psychiatric problems.

A Questionnaire to Rate Your Mindfulness

WITH PRACTICE, ALL of us can become more comfortable with meditation so that it becomes a part of our daily routine, not something you have to even think about. Believe me, mindfulness is easy. It may take time, but it does not take effort. It also takes patience and gentleness with yourself because you will no doubt encounter some discomfort as you try to make this part of your new routine. Relax and trust that it will become easier—eventually you'll look forward to it and miss it when you skip it—just like movement!

But for now, it's important to understand where you're at, just how mindful you are. Dr. Ruth Baer, a psychologist at the University of Kentucky, has developed a questionnaire that tracks how mindful you are in five different ways. She calls these the "five facets" of mindfulness, and they include:

1.   Your ability to *observe your thoughts*
2.   Your ability to *describe your thoughts* and feelings
3.   Your ability to *act with awareness* and stay present
4.   Your ability to *be nonjudgmental* of your own experience
5.   Your ability to *not react* when you feel intense emotions

Rate each of the following statements using the scale provided. Choose the response that best describes your own opinion of what is generally true for you.

MINDFULNESS QUESTIONNAIRE

Respond to each of the statements that best describes *your own opinion* of what is *generally true for you.* At the end of the questionnaire, add up the points according to the five facet categories of mindfulness.

1.   When I'm walking, I deliberately notice the sensations of my body moving.
- ( ) (1) Never or very rarely true
- ( ) (2) Rarely true
- ( ) (3) Sometimes true
- ( ) (4) Often true
- ( ) (5) Very often or always true

2.   I'm good at finding words to describe my feelings.
- ( ) (1) Never or very rarely true
- ( ) (2) Rarely true
- ( ) (3) Sometimes true
- ( ) (4) Often true
- ( ) (5) Very often or always true

3. I criticize myself for having irrational or inappropriate emotions.

○ (5) Never or very rarely true
○ (4) Rarely true
○ (3) Sometimes true
○ (2) Often true
○ (1) Very often or always true

4. I perceive my feelings and
emotions without having to
react to them.

○ (1) Never or very rarely true
○ (2) Rarely true
○ (3) Sometimes true
○ (4) Often true
○ (5) Very often or always true

5. When I do things, my mind wan-
ders off and I'm easily distracted.

○ (5) Never or very rarely true
○ (4) Rarely true
○ (3) Sometimes true
○ (2) Often true
○ (1) Very often or always true

6. When I take a shower or bath,
I stay alert to the sensations
of water on my body.

○ (1) Never or very rarely true
○ (2) Rarely true
○ (3) Sometimes true
○ (4) Often true
○ (5) Very often or always true

7. I can easily put my beliefs,
opinions, and expectations
into words.

○ (1) Never or very rarely true
○ (2) Rarely true
○ (3) Sometimes true
○ (4) Often true
○ (5) Very often or always true

8. I don't pay attention to what I'm
doing because I'm daydreaming,
worrying, or otherwise distracted.

○ (5) Never or very rarely true
○ (4) Rarely true
○ (3) Sometimes true
○ (2) Often true
○ (1) Very often or always true

9. I watch my feelings without
getting lost in them.

○ (1) Never or very rarely true
○ (2) Rarely true
○ (3) Sometimes true
○ (4) Often true
○ (5) Very often or always true

10. I tell myself I shouldn't be
feeling the way I'm feeling.

○ (5) Never or very rarely true
○ (4) Rarely true
○ (3) Sometimes true
○ (2) Often true
○ (1) Very often or always true

11. I notice how foods and drinks affect my thoughts, bodily sensations, and emotions.
   - ○ (1) Never or very rarely true
   - ○ (2) Rarely true
   - ○ (3) Sometimes true
   - ○ (4) Often true
   - ○ (5) Very often or always true

12. It's hard for me to find the words to describe what I'm thinking.
   - ○ (5) Never or very rarely true
   - ○ (4) Rarely true
   - ○ (3) Sometimes true
   - ○ (2) Often true
   - ○ (1) Very often or always true

13. I am easily distracted.
   - ○ (5) Never or very rarely true
   - ○ (4) Rarely true
   - ○ (3) Sometimes true
   - ○ (2) Often true
   - ○ (1) Very often or always true

14. I believe some of my thoughts are abnormal or bad and I shouldn't think that way.
   - ○ (5) Never or very rarely true
   - ○ (4) Rarely true
   - ○ (3) Sometimes true
   - ○ (2) Often true
   - ○ (1) Very often or always true

15. I pay attention to sensations, such as the wind in my hair or sun on my face.
   - ○ (1) Never or very rarely true
   - ○ (2) Rarely true
   - ○ (3) Sometimes true
   - ○ (4) Often true
   - ○ (5) Very often or always true

16. I have trouble thinking of the right words to express how I feel about things.
   - ○ (5) Never or very rarely true
   - ○ (4) Rarely true
   - ○ (3) Sometimes true
   - ○ (2) Often true
   - ○ (1) Very often or always true

17. I make judgments about whether my thoughts are good or bad.
   - ○ (5) Never or very rarely true
   - ○ (4) Rarely true
   - ○ (3) Sometimes true
   - ○ (2) Often true
   - ○ (1) Very often or always true

18. I find it difficult to stay focused on what's happening in the present.
   - ○ (5) Never or very rarely true
   - ○ (4) Rarely true
   - ○ (3) Sometimes true
   - ○ (2) Often true
   - ○ (1) Very often or always true

19. When I have distressing thoughts or images, I "step back" and am aware of the thought or image without getting taken over by it.
   - ○ (1) Never or very rarely true
   - ○ (2) Rarely true
   - ○ (3) Sometimes true
   - ○ (4) Often true
   - ○ (5) Very often or always true

20. I pay attention to sounds, such as clocks ticking, birds chirping, or cars passing.
   - ○ (5) Never or very rarely true
   - ○ (4) Rarely true
   - ○ (3) Sometimes true
   - ○ (2) Often true
   - ○ (1) Very often or always true

21. In difficult situations, I can pause without immediately reacting.
   - ○ (1) Never or very rarely true
   - ○ (2) Rarely true
   - ○ (3) Sometimes true
   - ○ (4) Often true
   - ○ (5) Very often or always true

22. When I have a sensation in my body, it's difficult for me to describe it because I can't find the right words.
   - ○ (5) Never or very rarely true
   - ○ (4) Rarely true
   - ○ (3) Sometimes true
   - ○ (2) Often true
   - ○ (1) Very often or always true

23. It seems I am "running on automatic" without much awareness of what I'm doing.
   - ○ (5) Never or very rarely true
   - ○ (4) Rarely true
   - ○ (3) Sometimes true
   - ○ (2) Often true
   - ○ (1) Very often or always true

24. When I have distressing thoughts or images, I feel calm soon after.
   - ○ (1) Never or very rarely true
   - ○ (2) Rarely true
   - ○ (3) Sometimes true
   - ○ (4) Often true
   - ○ (5) Very often or always true

25. I tell myself that I shouldn't be thinking the way I'm thinking.
   - ○ (5) Never or very rarely true
   - ○ (4) Rarely true
   - ○ (3) Sometimes true
   - ○ (2) Often true
   - ○ (1) Very often or always true

26. I notice the smells and aromas around me.
   - ○ (1) Never or very rarely true
   - ○ (2) Rarely true
   - ○ (3) Sometimes true
   - ○ (4) Often true
   - ○ (5) Very often or always true

27. Even when I'm feeling terribly upset, I can find a way to put it into words.
- ○ (1) Never or very rarely true
- ○ (2) Rarely true
- ○ (3) Sometimes true
- ○ (4) Often true
- ○ (5) Very often or always true

28. I rush through activities without being really attentive to them.
- ○ (5) Never or very rarely true
- ○ (4) Rarely true
- ○ (3) Sometimes true
- ○ (2) Often true
- ○ (1) Very often or always true

29. When I have distressing thoughts or images I am able just to notice them without reacting.
- ○ (1) Never or very rarely true
- ○ (2) Rarely true
- ○ (3) Sometimes true
- ○ (4) Often true
- ○ (5) Very often or always true

30. I think some of my emotions are bad or inappropriate and I shouldn't feel them.
- ○ (5) Never or very rarely true
- ○ (4) Rarely true
- ○ (3) Sometimes true
- ○ (2) Often true
- ○ (1) Very often or always true

31. I notice visual elements in art or nature, such as colors, shapes, textures, or patterns of light and shadow.
- ○ (1) Never or very rarely true
- ○ (2) Rarely true
- ○ (3) Sometimes true
- ○ (4) Often true
- ○ (5) Very often or always true

32. My natural tendency is to put my experiences into words.
- ○ (1) Never or very rarely true
- ○ (2) Rarely true
- ○ (3) Sometimes true
- ○ (4) Often true
- ○ (5) Very often or always true

33. When I have distressing thoughts or images, I just notice them and let them go.
- ○ (1) Never or very rarely true
- ○ (2) Rarely true
- ○ (3) Sometimes true
- ○ (4) Often true
- ○ (5) Very often or always true

34. I do jobs or tasks automatically without being aware of what I'm doing.
- ○ (5) Never or very rarely true
- ○ (4) Rarely true
- ○ (3) Sometimes true
- ○ (2) Often true
- ○ (1) Very often or always true

35. When I have distressing thoughts or images, I judge myself as good or bad, depending what the thought/image is about.

  ○ (5) Never or very rarely true
  ○ (4) Rarely true
  ○ (3) Sometimes true
  ○ (2) Often true
  ○ (1) Very often or always true

36. I pay attention to how my emotions affect my thoughts and behavior.

  ○ (1) Never or very rarely true
  ○ (2) Rarely true
  ○ (3) Sometimes true
  ○ (4) Often true
  ○ (5) Very often or always true

37. I can usually describe how I feel at the moment in considerable detail.

  ○ (1) Never or very rarely true
  ○ (2) Rarely true
  ○ (3) Sometimes true
  ○ (4) Often true
  ○ (5) Very often or always true

38. I find myself doing things without paying attention.

  ○ (5) Never or very rarely true
  ○ (4) Rarely true
  ○ (3) Sometimes true
  ○ (2) Often true
  ○ (1) Very often or always true

39. I disapprove of myself when I have irrational ideas.

  ○ (5) Never or very rarely true
  ○ (4) Rarely true
  ○ (3) Sometimes true
  ○ (2) Often true
  ○ (1) Very often or always true

SCORING INFORMATION

The mindfulness questionnaire focuses on the five facets of mindfulness, which include:

✳ Your ability to be aware of and *observe* stimuli using your five senses.
✳ Your facility for identifying and *describing* your thoughts and feelings and putting them into words.
✳ Your tendency to *act while being aware* of your thoughts and feelings.
✳ Your likelihood of being *nonjudgmental* of your own behavior, thoughts, and feelings.
✳ Your ability to *not react* in response to thoughts and feelings.

Like anything, mindfulness takes practice to develop strength—knowing that some days will always be easier than others.

In order to determine your mindfulness score, total each of the five facets, then divide by the number of questions to get your score:

✳ For observation: questions 1, 6, 11, 15, 20, 26, 31, 36
Low score 1 to 2; medium 3 to 5; high 6 to 8

✳ For description: questions 2, 7, 12, 16, 22, 27, 32, 37
Low score 1 to 2; medium 3 to 5; high 6 to 8

✳ For acting with awareness: questions 5, 8, 13, 18, 23, 28, 34, 38
Low score 1 to 2; medium 3 to 5; high 6 to 8

✳ For nonjudgment: questions 3, 10, 14, 17, 25, 30, 35, 39
Low score 1 to 2; medium 3 to 5; high 6 to 8

✳ For nonreaction: questions 4, 9, 19, 21, 24, 29, 33
Low score 1 to 2; medium 3 to 5; high 6 to 7

When you tally your score in each of the five areas, consider where you are and how you might help yourself become more mindful. Don't judge yourself. Don't criticize yourself. Just honor and accept where you are now, knowing that the more often you practice meditation, the stronger you will get in these areas.

TYPES OF MEDITATION

Meditation has been practiced for thousands of years in many different cultures, especially in Indian, Chinese, and Christian traditions. Here are a few of the major types. (My favorites are TM and Kundalini.)

* Buddhist or Zen meditation (*zazen*)
* Vipassana
* Mindfulness meditation
* Insight meditation
* Loving-kindness meditation
* Mantra meditation
* Kundalini
* Transcendental meditation (TM)
* Contemplative prayer
* Chakra meditation
* Guided meditation

Recently, a number of really good meditation apps have become available for easy download to any device. Here is a list of my favorites.

* Headspace
* Omvana
* Simply Being
* Sitting Still
* Relax Melodies
* Buddhify
* Meditation Timer Pro
* The Mindfulness App
* Calm
* Smiling Mind

These apps offer different ways to enjoy meditation—listening to melodic music, following a guide through different breathing exercises, or guided meditative "tours" that move from focused attention to open monitoring. Many of them are free, so download now!

Begin at the Beginning

THOUGH THERE ARE many traditions and ways to approach meditation, they all share one thing in common: they begin with the breath. This connection to our breath is literally one of the most profound ways we can heal ourselves from stress, unease, and even disease.

Because we are generally addicted to complexity and busyness, reaching a state of authentic relaxation is a challenge. Many of us are locked into worry, hurry, and overwork and live on a kind of unaware autopilot that blocks out our ability to relax and become aware. I'm going to share a simple mindfulness practice that I do, as well as other ways to incorporate meditation (or meditative-like experiences) into your life so that all you've been doing—nurturing your intuitive relationship with yourself, eating clean, and moving so you feel alive—will be enhanced.

Here's what I do:

* I get out my iPhone.
* I set my timer for ten minutes.
* I sit cross-legged so I stay aware of my body. (If you have a bad back, sit on a chair. Lying down is also a good way to start because you will feel relaxed.)
* I start with three big breaths—in though my nose, out through my mouth.
* Then after the three big breaths, just breathe through my nose.
* Then I pick a color—and focus on the color with my eyes closed.
* I let thoughts come in and simply observe them, watching them drift.
* If I get distracted, I refocus with my breath and chosen color.
* When the timer goes off, I gently open my eyes and sit, absorbing the light.
* When I have time, I go to my Drawing Board and write down all the thoughts that came to me during the meditation. This last step can cue me in to what was distracting me. Was it an old boyfriend? Worries

about finances? My work schedule? Then, with intention, I put aside these thoughts in a conscious way.

* Next, I write down whether the meditation was great and I feel clear— or if it was difficult. I try to rate my experience on a scale of 1 to 5, 5 being fantastic and 1 being very difficult.

This whole process takes about ten minutes total and helps me create more awareness of my thoughts and feelings and where I am in my life. It also helps me set intentions: sometimes I remember I haven't called someone back, or that I need to be more patient with my kids, or that I need to stop judging myself or others.

DRAWING BOARD

Everyone has at least one great teacher in their life; mine is my mom. This is one of her favorite meditations.

"At times when I feel spent, flitting from one thought to the next, I just sit myself down and meditate. I sit in silence, take three cleansing breaths with a smile on my face, feel the weight of my body relaxing on my cushion, and then visualize my heart beating in my chest. I focus there for some time, holding the energy with loving kindness, nurturing the love and preciousness of life. Sometimes it's an emotional release. I have gone inside. I feel home. After five minutes, I focus on my breath as it quiets and slows down, and then continue for another five minutes. Sometimes I stay there longer, letting my invading thoughts float away like clouds, and return to my breathing.

"I then see my children in front of me, and shed light and gratitude on them for allowing me to be the vessel lucky enough to bring them to life, to give them the chance to flourish in this world as separate, beautiful human beings, and I surround them with light and deep love. Upon opening my eyes, I feel refreshed and joyful. My frenzied mind is calm, and I am back in tune with what matters most: Love."

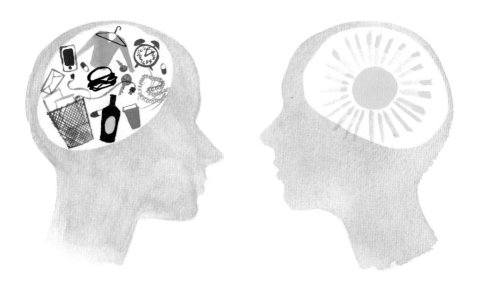

It's Not Just About You

ONE OF THE most fascinating things I learned from my own meditation practice is how it affects other people. When I meditate on a regular basis, my relationships with others become warmer and steadier, and I feel more trusting. In fact, neuroscientists and psychologists have determined that there are many ways that meditating can positively affect all of our relationships—with children, siblings, adult parents, coworkers, and friends.

1. You don't overreact.

    When we are stressed, it's easy for us to get impatient or angry and lose our tempers. Think of arriving home after a long day at work or travel. You're bombarded at the front door by what your kids need—papers signed, help with homework, a fight over a favorite toy—or an off-the-cuff remark that your partner might lob at you. Instead of barking back or getting hurt, a more mindful person will not react with anger or frustration. You will resist getting swept up in someone else's emotional situation.

2. You will become more emotionally flexible and not stay stuck in bad moods.
Mindfulness training enables you to see your emotions more objectively. Instead of being pulled down into a dark mood, regardless of the trigger, you will catch yourself and shift your mood more consciously. You will feel more in control of your moods rather than swept up by them. This will help you save more positive energy for your interactions with others, especially those close to you, whom we tend to project onto most often.

3. You will become a better listener.
With increased ability to focus, you become calmer and more able to listen and tune in to other people. Scientists have also seen an increase in people's intuition—you will take in that unspoken information and trust your gut more often.

4. You will become more empathetic.
Instead of being able to relate only to someone whose situation is similar to your own, you will be more able to put yourself in someone else's shoes and really connect to another person's experience.

5. You will more likely be compassionate and kind toward others.
The research on mindfulness shows that when people learn to meditate regularly, they become more broadly compassionate, more likely to act on their beliefs and ideals, and demonstrate greater interest in the social good. It's like having a healthier relationship with your whole community, not just the people closest to you.

Meditation has also made me a more patient parent, and more aware of how I bring my own stresses into the home or my boys' lives. I'm not perfect every day, but meditation gives me the direction and energy to quickly refocus if I do get impatient with them. Meditation also helps me be more communicative with my kids. Since I am more aware of how I am feeling, I don't react. I take a minute and am able to frame the situation for them. If I'm particularly stressed or tired, I'll say something like, "Mommy doesn't feel so good today—I've feeling really stressed, so let's all be aware of that." This lets the boys know that I need them to be more aware and it helps me control my emotional state—it's a win-win for everyone!

I truly believe that meditation soothes the soul, unburdens the mind, and supports the body. I hope you find the joy!

I truly believe that meditation soothes the soul, unburdens the mind, and supports the body. I hope you find the joy!

CHAPTER SEVEN

THE PURIFYING CLEANSE

I HAVE A CONFESSION: I love to cleanse. I love the ritual of taking the toxins out of my body, resetting my metabolism, and restoring a deep calm and balance. And that's the purpose of a cleanse: to get rid of toxins and the buildup of waste products that our organs—the liver, the kidneys, and the colon—can't get rid of on their own. Like sludge, this leftover waste slows down our digestion, hampers our immune systems, and often causes us to gain weight.

Cleanses are not meant to be a weekly routine or a way to diet—no matter what form, a cleanse is not a sustainable way to eat. But done in the right way, at the right time, a cleanse can be a wonderful way to reinvigorate your body and your mind. Cleanses can also help you break the cycle of bad habits and give yourself a fresh start.

I do two primary cleanses twice a year—a seven- to ten-day cleanse in the spring and another in the fall. But any time I feel sluggish, or my body feels out of balance if I've been working lots of long hours, traveling a lot, or if I just feel worn down and about to get sick, I do a short mini-cleanse of one to three days. At the end of a cleanse, I feel clearheaded, lighter, and more energetic. So consider a cleanse the next time you want that reset to happen in a quick, intense way! Here are some options, but remember, there is no half-assing a cleanse—long or short, you've got to go for it, and you can't cheat!

Three Simple Cleanses

FOR ME, A cleanse can be relatively complex and long (seven to ten days) or easy and short (one to three days). The simplest cleanse is an elimination cleanse, in which you take out one or more of the three most troubling foods:

1. Gluten
2. Dairy
3. Sugar

Although there has been a lot of discussion about the rise in gluten intolerance, scientists, nutritionists, and educators agree that gluten, the protein in grains, has changed its molecular form and is now much harder to digest for most people. You don't have to have celiac disease or have been diagnosed with gluten sensitivity to overreact to gluten. That's my situation. By and large, I have stopped eating bread and most wheat flour unless it's an artisanal bread made from non-GMO flour. That probably sounds fairly snooty, but I've got to be honest here: Without the gluten in my diet, I have so much more energy and all the puffiness in my face, belly, and neck disappears.

Without the gluten in my diet, I have so much more energy and all the puffiness in my face, belly, and neck disappears.

Dairy is another food group that has changed a lot in recent years. I think I partially grew up on ice cream. I could eat cartons and cartons and didn't know how to stop. The sweet coolness in my mouth, the satisfying slide down my throat—all so delicious. But as I've gotten older, my body cannot tolerate much dairy. Occasionally, I indulge in yogurt (in a smoothie or frozen) or hard cheeses, but gone is the half-and-half in my coffee and the milk in my tea. Taking out dairy is known to rapidly balance blood sugar (did you know that milk has a lot of sugar in it?) and help facilitate weight loss.

Finally, the worst offender of all: sugar. If there is one thing we can all do without, it truly is sugar. Sugar messes with our digestion and our ability to metabolize fat, produces chronic inflammation (an overreaction by the body's immune system that contributes to many diseases including heart disease, Crohn's disease, arthritis, diabetes, and some cancers) throughout the body, and causes weight gain. Sugar is a villain like no other. And when you remove sugar from your diet, all of those systems calm down. Your digestion perks up; you begin to use up stored fat, and inflammation in your gut lining calms down. But quitting sugar is not easy. Most of us have an addictive relationship with sugar and find it hard to resist cravings. If that sounds familiar, check out page 173 for more on how to tame the sugar menace.

A next-level cleanse would be a juice or hot broth cleanse. This is one to three days when you ingest only liquids. This is the idea behind the popular Master Cleanse brand of products. The challenge with these is that you will eventually need to eat, so approach this type of cleanse for only a short amount of time.

VEGETABLE DETOX BROTH

When I do a quick one-day broth cleanse, I use this vegetable detox broth, which is easy on your body's digestive system and also loaded with wonderful vitamins and minerals. I sip on this throughout the day.

2 medium carrots, chopped

3 celery stalks, cut into thirds

2 large garlic cloves, finely chopped

½ bunch kale, leaves only (be sure to take off the stems, which are what makes kale so bitter)

½ butternut squash, peeled and chopped

¼ cup fresh parsley, chopped

½ ounce fresh ginger, peeled and chopped

½ teaspoon ground turmeric

½ teaspoon sea salt

¼ teaspoon freshly ground black pepper

3 quarts filtered water

1. Place all the ingredients in a heavy pot, slow cooker, or stockpot.
2. Cover and bring to a boil, then reduce the heat and simmer for 3 to 4 hours.
3. Enjoy as is, or strain and enjoy as broth!

CLEANSES ARE NOT DIETS

It's crucial to understand that cleanses are not meant to be sustained. Have I tried a juice cleanse? A raw-food cleanse? A water with lemon juice and apple cider vinegar cleanse? Guilty of all charges! But that is no way to eat or live. Do a cleanse when you are stuck in a rut and want to detox your body and mind, not when you want to drop a quick eight pounds.

Are You Addicted to Sugar?

TAKE THIS SHORT quiz.

✳ Do you eat when you're not hungry?

✳ Do you experience a "food coma" after eating?

✳ Do you feel bad about your eating habits or avoid certain activities because of your eating?

✳ Do you get withdrawal symptoms if you cut down on or stop eating sugar or flour?

✳ Do you need more and more of the same bad foods just to feel good?

If you answered yes to any of these, then it's more than likely you have an addictive relationship with sugar and could benefit from a sugar detox. See my suggestion below!

Taming the Sugar Menace Cleanse

YOU PROBABLY KNOW this already: sugar wreaks havoc on your system. If you have an addictive relationship with sugar or eat more than 40 grams of sugar a day, it's probably a good idea to detox from sugar. Look at your Drawing Board and list of foods you've been eating for the past few days. Circle those foods that contain sugar. Add up (or estimate) the amount of sugar you consumed over a three- to four-day period. If it tops 40 grams, then you might want to consider a sugar detox.

Try this strategy for two or three days and see how you feel. If you feel remarkably better (you're sleeping better, your cravings and mood swings calm down, and your skin clears up), chances are you have too much sugar in your system. These six tips will help you get rid of the excess sugar in your system while also balancing your blood sugar. If after two to three days you feel remarkably better, continue until you've reached five full days. If you still feel remarkably better, stick to it for another two days. Remember to keep a record of how you feel in your Drawing Board. This record will help remind you of how low you used to feel when you were controlled by sugar—and how good you feel after you removed from your diet the sugar-laden foods that are making you sick.

1. Ideally, for five days avoid any foods that contain added sugar; this typically means any food that comes in a box, package, or a can (or anything that has a label). Stick to real, whole, fresh food.

2. Take away any beverages that contain added sugar, high-fructose corn syrup, or artificial sweeteners (artificial sweeteners trigger a similar insulin response, so you need to stay away from diet anything!).

3. Sugary drinks are the single biggest source of sugar calories in our diet. This includes sodas, juices other than green vegetable juice, sports drinks, and sweetened teas or coffees. One twenty-ounce soda has fifteen tea-spoons of sugar; Gatorade contains fourteen teaspoons of sugar in one eight-ounce bottle.

4. Increase your lean protein intake and include it at every meal. Protein will dampen your sugar craving and help you feel satisfied. Start the day with eggs or a protein shake. Include nuts, seeds, eggs, fish, chicken, or grass-fed meat for protein in every meal. A serving size is four to six ounces, or the size of your palm.

5. Up your veggies. Veggies also help you kill the sugar cravings.

6. Make sure to get your good fat in. Fat doesn't make you fat, sugar does. Fat makes you full, balances your blood sugar, and is necessary for fueling your

cells. Along with protein, make sure to include good fats at every meal and snack, including nuts and seeds (which also contain protein), extra-virgin olive oil, coconut butter, avocados, and omega-3 fats from fish. Again, the fuller you feel, the less likely you will crave the sugar.

7.   Stay away from alcohol. This may be obvious, but wine, liquor, and even beer contain sugar, which can trigger all those cravings we are trying to banish. So give yourself a week and skip the glass of wine!

By the end of a week, you will feel not only more clearheaded but lighter and calmer.

A Three-Day Ayurvedic Cleanse

AYURVEDIC PHYSICIANS RECOMMEND a cleanse at the change of every season, especially going into fall and into spring, as a way to refresh the immune system and get rid of the buildup that any diet, no matter what you eat and where you live, will bring.

In Ayurvedic philosophy, good, healthy functioning of our physical-emotional-mental system begins with proper digestion, absorption, and elimination of our food—all of which comprises our metabolism. If these processes are impaired or are not working up to snuff, then our bodies become vulnerable to disease. For Ayurvedics, a cleanse strengthens our metabolic energy, or *agni* (which means "fire" in Sanskrit).

Different from what we typically associate with cleanses (water and lemon, apple cider vinegar, or juices), Ayurvedic cleanses are much more moderate—and filling! You never get hungry! Why? Because you eat a lot—but of a simple dish called *kitchari* that is made up of a blend of basmati rice, mung beans, and spices. It is tasty, filling, and is easy to digest, helping you clear the digestive tract of toxins and restore balance in the gut.

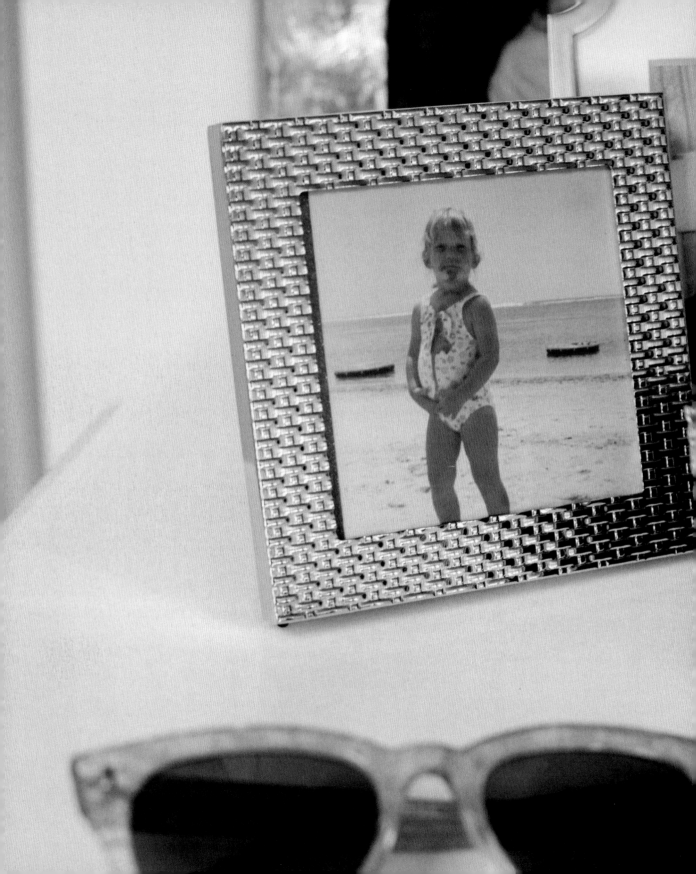

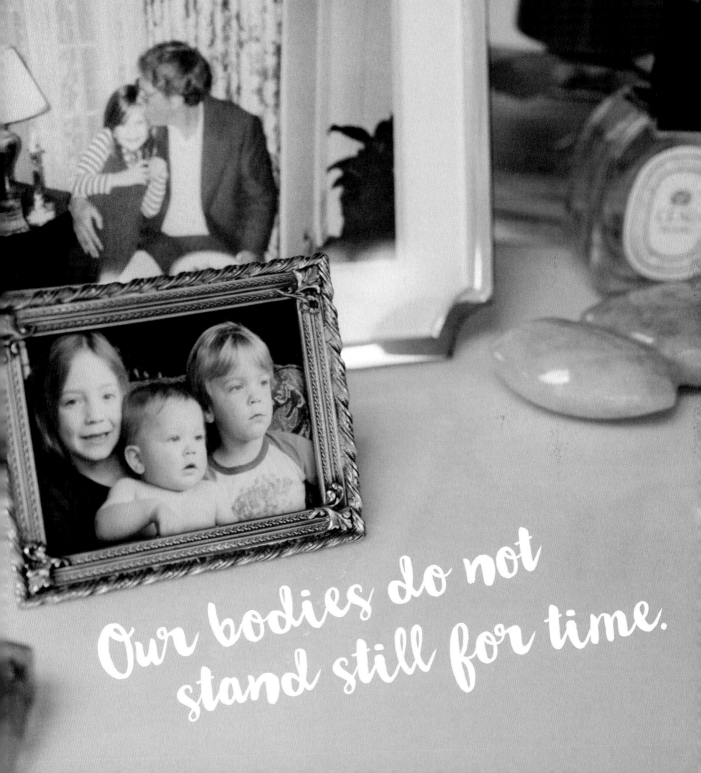

Our bodies do not stand still for time.

These cleanses go for three days, so you need to prepare ahead of time. This means shopping and having all of your supplies on hand. Tell someone close to you that you're doing this cleanse so that you have support and someone else to hold you accountable when things get tough—and believe me, they will! You also need to prepare emotionally. Stuff comes up during cleanses. Take it from me. Old stuff that you thought was long in the past. You will be releasing held energy and old hurts. The release you feel is your body thanking you for this time of self-care.

You will be releasing held energy and old hurts. The release you feel is your body thanking you for this time of self-care.

The good news is that these feelings are being released, which means you can wave good-bye to them. On the other hand, they are tough to get through. It's therefore really important that you keep your Drawing Board nearby at all times so you can keep a record of all that you're experiencing. You might also want to add an extra meditation to your day during the cleanse.

To do this cleanse, you need some simple Indian cooking staples (listed on page 180) so that you have everything you need to start the kitchari cleanse.

Technically, to do the cleanse all you need to do is eat kitchari (or steel-cut oatmeal) and drink the lemon-ginger detox tea along with plenty of water.

Here's the schedule:

* The evening before you start the cleanse, you will want to prepare your kitchari for the following day.
* When you wake up, scrape your tongue with a tongue scraper, if you have one. (They are quite inexpensive, and I suggest purchasing one for your cleanse!) If you are new to tongue scraping, be sure to scrape from the back of your tongue, right where the bumpy section of your

tongue (where your taste buds live) ends. When I first started scraping my tongue, I accidentally clipped a taste bud, which hurts quite a bit!

✳ Do a gentle stretch or some yoga to open up the body before you eat.

✳ Sit down and mindfully enjoy either a warm bowl of kitchari or steel-cut oatmeal. Feel free to add spices such as cinnamon or cardamom. (Don't add fruit!)

✳ For the remainder of the day, eat as much kitchari as you wish, whenever you're hungry, but try not to stuff yourself. Sip on your lemon-ginger tea or water between meals.

✳ Try to eat your final meal before seven p.m. to give plenty of time for digestion before sleep.

✳ Repeat this for three days. If you get very hungry or feel yourself with very low blood sugar, you can add some lean protein. And you can always eat as much kitchari as you like. This is not meant to be a weight-loss week. Its purpose is different.

Some of the early side effects of a cleanse are:

✳ Headaches

✳ Body aches

✳ Irritability

✳ Fatigue

These are all normal reactions to the body getting rid of toxins. If you are experiencing these symptoms, make sure that you up your water intake to make sure that the toxins are being ushered out of the system.

KITCHARI

There are many recipes for kitchari; try this one and then sample some others! If you want to add more heft to your kitchari, simply add 2 cups of a liquefied blend of vegetables like asparagus, carrots, celery, green beans, summer squash, sweet potatoes, winter squash, or zucchini! Enjoy!

1 cup yellow mung beans
1 teaspoon grated fresh ginger
2 tablespoons unsweetened shredded coconut
3 tablespoons ghee or unsalted butter
½ teaspoon ground cinnamon
¼ teaspoon ground cardamom
¼ teaspoon freshly ground black pepper
¼ teaspoon ground cloves
¼ teaspoon ground turmeric
¼ teaspoon sea salt
3 bay leaves
1 cup white basmati rice
6 cups filtered water

1. Rinse the mung beans and let soak in water (enough to cover the beans) for 2 to 3 hours. Set aside.
2. In a blender, combine the ginger, coconut, and ½ cup water. Set aside.
3. In a large saucepan set over medium heat, melt the ghee. Add the cinnamon, cardamom, pepper, clove, turmeric, salt, and bay leaves and heat until warm, not boiling.
4. Drain the mung beans. Stir them into the spice mixture in the saucepan.
5. Add the rice to the saucepan. Stir in the blended spice and coconut mixture, followed by the water.
6. Bring to a boil, cover, and cook on low heat for 25 to 30 minutes, until soft. Remember to remove the bay leaves.

LEMON-GINGER DETOX TEA

Sipping on a detox tea as you cleanse can help strengthen the detox effect on all of your organs, as well as your digestive system. Here's one that I particularly enjoy!

1 (4-inch) piece fresh ginger

6 cups filtered water

2 cinnamon sticks

1 teaspoon ground turmeric

½ teaspoon cayenne pepper

1 teaspoon raw honey per mug

Squeeze of lemon juice per mug

1. Peel the ginger and slice it thinly on an angle. Use the side of the knife to smash the ginger (exposing more surface area).

2. In a large saucepan, combine the ginger slices and water and bring to a boil over high heat. Turn the heat to low and simmer for 10 minutes.

3. Add the cinnamon, turmeric, and cayenne and simmer for another 10 minutes.

4. Strain into a mug (you can refrigerate the rest to enjoy later).

5. Stir in the honey and lemon.

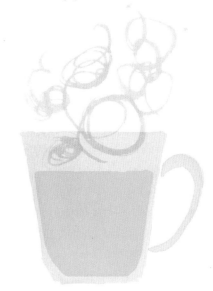

Cleanse and Rebalance Your Dosha

REMEMBER THE THREE body types, or doshas, of Ayurveda? These body types are reflections of our general physical, mental, and emotional constitutions and temperaments. A quick way to get your dosha back into balance is through a cleanse. See page 183 for a quick reminder of whether your dosha is out of balance—you might benefit from a cleanse!

Toxins to Avoid

IN ADDITION TO the toxins that can accumulate from eating processed foods, we are also vulnerable to taking in toxins from our immediate surroundings. Volumes of books could be written on modern-day toxic exposures, and while it may be impossible to list every possibility, if you avoid the most notorious offenders, you'll be way ahead of the game. In general, this includes tossing out your toxic household cleaners, personal hygiene products, air fresheners, bug sprays, lawn pesticides, and insecticides, just to name a few, and replacing them with nontoxic alternatives. In terms of specific toxins, some of the most hazardous yet commonly encountered ones include:

* Mercury—found in dental amalgams and fish.
* Fluoride—found in toothpaste, fluoridated water, and nonorganic food (due to the widespread use of fluoride-based pesticides. For example, conventionally grown iceberg lettuce can contain as much as 180 ppm of fluoride—180 times higher than what's recommended in drinking water).
* EMFs—Electromagnetic field exposures are becoming increasingly pervasive and they can interact unfavorably with your biology.

DOSHA	SYMPTOMS OF IMBALANCE
VATA WINTER/AIR AND ETHER 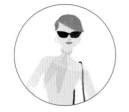	Dry or rough skin Insomnia Constipation Fatigue Headaches Intolerance of cold Underweight or losing weight Anxiety, worry, and restlessness Attention Deficit with Hyperactivity Disorder
PITTA SUMMER/FIRE AND WATER 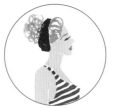	Rashes Inflammatory skin conditions (including acne) Stomachaches Diarrhea Controlling and manipulative behavior Visual problems or burning in the eyes Excessive body heat Hostility, irritability Excessive competitive drive
KAPHA SPRING/EARTH AND WATER 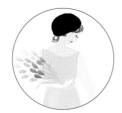	Oily skin Slow digestion Sinus congestion Nasal allergies Asthma Obesity Skin growths Possessiveness, neediness Apathy Depression Difficulty paying attention

* Bisphenol-A (BPA) and Bisphenol-S (BPS)—Used in the manufacture of polycarbonate plastics, bisphenols are estrogen-mimicking chemicals that can leach into food or drinks from the plastic containers holding them. These chemicals are known to be particularly dangerous for pregnant women, infants, and children.

* To avoid plastic toxins such as bisphenols, opt for glass over plastic, especially when it comes to products that will come into contact with food or beverages, or those intended for pregnant women, infants, and children. This applies to canned goods as well, which are a major source of BPA (and possibly other chemicals) exposure, so whenever you can, choose jarred goods over canned goods, or opt for fresh instead. Another good idea is to ditch plastic teething toys for your little ones and choose natural wood or fabric varieties instead.

* Phthalates—found in soft plastics such as polyvinyl chloride (PVC), as well as many toiletries, including shampoos, toothpastes, and cosmetics. Phthalates are one of the most pervasive types of endocrine-disrupting chemicals discovered so far and have been linked to a wide range of developmental and reproductive "gender-bending" effects.

Great Detox Tools:
Saunas, Steam Baths, and Whirlpools

STEAM BATHS, SAUNAS, and hot tubs can also be a simple yet effective way to detox and an enjoyable addition to your cleanse. The heat and moisture not only help tissues relax, but the overall process can enhance your metabolism and circulation, and help oxygenate your tissues so that you feel more balanced.

Since our skin is a major organ of elimination, sweating out the toxins can help us detox—especially if you don't sweat on a regular basis. Wearing certain synthetic materials, staying outside in the sun too often for long periods of time, and being too sedentary can all weaken your skin's ability to get rid of toxic buildup. Steam baths are great for detoxifying your water-based organs. So if you have lung, kidney, or bladder problems—respiratory congestion, bladder or kidney infections, or the tendency to develop kidney stones—a steam bath with some essential oil can also be beneficial.

Whirlpools or Jacuzzis are recommended for lymphatic and neurological problems, including swollen glands or any nervous system disorders ranging from back pain to carpal tunnel syndrome. However, you'll want to make sure it's not loaded full of chlorine and other harmful chemicals, as that will defeat the whole purpose. Ideally, you'll also want to use filtered water to avoid as many contaminants as possible.

If you've never taken a sauna before, you want to spend only a few minutes in there—about four minutes tops. Then, for each subsequent sauna, add about thirty seconds, and slowly work your way up to somewhere between fifteen and thirty minutes. The reason for this is because the detoxification process can in some cases be severe, depending on your toxic load.

The Emotional Side to Cleansing

KNOW THIS: WHEN you rid your body of toxins and other sludge, a lot of old emotions that are stored in our bodies come to the surface. As Dr. Richard Anderson explains in his book *Cleanse and Purify Thyself,* "emotions get trapped in cells and when we fast or cleanse, these emotion-carrying cells, especially weak, dead, or dying cells are rapidly released from the body. In this way we release forever the emotions that were trapped within those cells." It's important to be mindful and let yourself be open to these often negative, highly charged emotions.

* First, allow the feelings to happen. Don't resist or mask them.
* Second, observe your feelings and try to identify them. Sad, angry, embarrassed, ashamed.

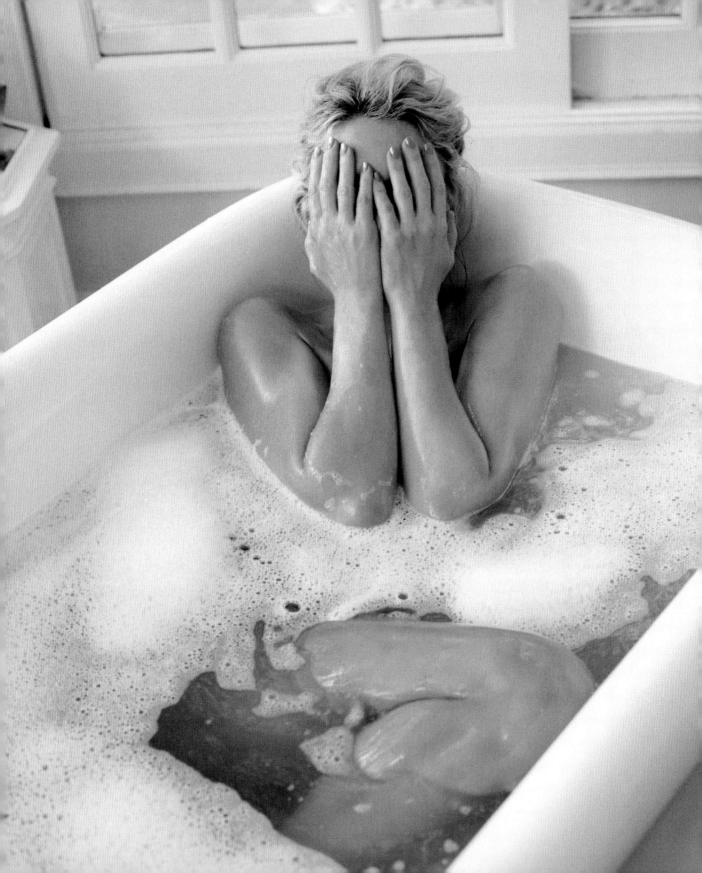

* Third, can you identify the origin of the feelings? Are they associated with a specific experience, event, or trauma?
* Fourth, lean in to your support system. Don't go it alone. Share your experience; it will lighten your load.
* Finally, give yourself some pleasure—what activities do you enjoy doing? What sensations might give you pleasure?

Again, making a record of this experience in your Drawing Board will increase your self-awareness and your connection to your mind and body. The more aware you are, the less surprised you will be when stress begins to wear on you. You will also have more resilience when times get tough. For me, the combination of cleansing and meditation provides powerful protection and helps me feel centered and happy.

One time, I got dumped. Yup. Out of the blue, this guy I'd been dating told me it was over. At the time, the news completely blindsided me and I was overwhelmed. My heart was broken. My go-to person, my mom, immediately told me to cleanse.

"What? My heart is broken, not my body! What is a cleanse going to help?! That's the last thing I need!"

"Trust me." That's all she said.

So I began a ten-day cleanse that was pretty intense. I have to admit that the first four days were a disaster—I was a mess. Then I began to turn the corner. I began to realize that though I felt incredibly vulnerable and shocked, all my intense emotions and feelings had nothing to do with the guy. The feelings that were surfacing were tied to old stuff. Suddenly I realized that I wasn't focused on the guy at all. I was too focused on the intensity of my own experience.

The next few days were all about letting go. I was letting go of my attachment to old situations, old ways of reacting, and old ways of feeling ashamed. He barely crossed my mind.

What can I say? Thanks to a cleanse, I was happy to get dumped!

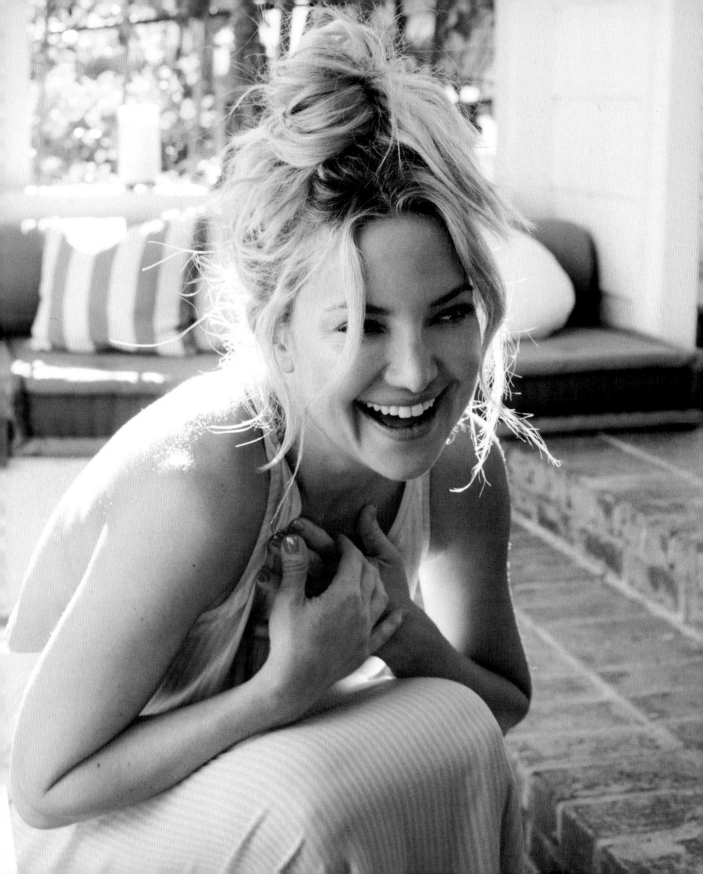

CHAPTER EIGHT

FINDING PRETTY HAPPY

*"Happiness is not something ready-made.
It comes from your own actions."*

—DALAI LAMA

LATELY WE'VE HEARD a lot about happiness—the science of happiness, how you can "find" happiness, how you can stumble upon happiness, and how you can become even 10 percent happier and feel a lot better in your life. All of these articles and books have intrigued me (as I've mentioned, I love self-help books; they act as my ongoing back-to-school journey). But I am not simply echoing the bunnymen here. I've spent a lot of time and a lot of energy soul searching, asking and continuing to ask myself questions, and truly observing my everyday experience. It's been a journey fueled by curiosity: Where is all this taking me? What does it mean to me? What's the point? And am I having fun yet?

To me, *happiness* is one of those words that is not an idea, it's an experience. You've got to figure it out from the inside, and no one can tell you how to be happy. But I do think that what most of us experience as happiness is a combination of three things: being able to experience pleasure in a spontaneous, playful, sensual way; being content with what we have in life and staying present and grateful; and getting in touch with what matters most.

I may not have all the answers; in fact, I hope I don't, because I don't ever want to stop learning and feeding my curiosity. But I have realized that through my mindfulness practice; through eating cleaner, healthier, whole foods; and staying connected to my body in a physical and emotional way, that I am actually pretty happy. I am also having much more fun—a regular glutton for pleasure! I'm no longer waiting for a job to be finished, my kids to get a teensy bit older, or my mood to change. I've figured out that having pleasure and enjoyment in my life makes a huge impact on how I experience everything—from parenting to work and everything in between.

I'm also more content. I rarely get stuck in that place of "I wish I had." I am much more comfortable in "I'm so lucky I have." This shift in attitude might sound simple, but it actually requires subtle yet very concrete adjustments in how I think and act on a day-to-day basis.

So this chapter is all about offering some of my insights into how I made the shift—how slight tweaks have made a big difference in how I wake up in the morning and how I deal with myself and other people in my life. I also have noticed that I feel more comfortable, not as frazzled or up and down as I used to feel. I don't get caught up in worries about my kids or work; I don't fixate on things beyond my control—like if my next film will be X, Y, or Z. I kind of go with the flow, trusting that all is well. Don't get me wrong—I can still sit up for hours with my girlfriends and talk about boys and relationships and work and kids—girls love to dwell and fixate on things until we fix them—I still indulge in all the normal things that become loops in our brains. *My kids are driving me crazy! I have so much to do!* I don't judge myself when I'm cranky or irritable or too tired to work out. I don't judge others who don't live the way I do and make different choices.

I let myself enjoy life—being with my children and family, diving into a new film project, going on a long hike in the canyon by my house. I connect with my sensuality and sexuality in ways that make me feel vibrant and alive. This connection to pleasure is a lifeline of energy for me and provides another antidote to stress.

But ultimately the pleasure and the contentment drive me to what matters most—my family. Of course I take my work and career seriously. I want to succeed and make a contribution in whatever way I can. My health matters to me. But at the end of the day (actually, at the very beginning of each day), I always remind myself of the people in my life whom I love. My children, my brothers, my parents—they motivate me in all the other areas. I think that's the best we can do: stay aware of who and what matters most in our lives, make sure we relax enough to play and give ourselves some kick-back fun, and strive for that middle ground of contentment—where what we do and have satisfies us.

Rediscovering Pleasure

ON THE ONE hand it may seem like our society is addicted to pleasure—we are constantly reminded of ways to feel good, relax, and take the edge off—gambling in casinos, advertisements for vacations, and, of course, the inundation of information about sex—when to have it, how often to have it, and "here, take this pill so you can have it." Yet despite this frenzy of stimulation, most people seem to have a hard time relaxing enough to ever experience pleasure. I was in the same boat when I had my first son. I was only twenty-three and completely overwhelmed by all that motherhood encompassed. It was as if overnight I forgot to have fun. I was always worrying about Ryder's feeding schedule, nap schedule, and whether I was being a good enough mother!

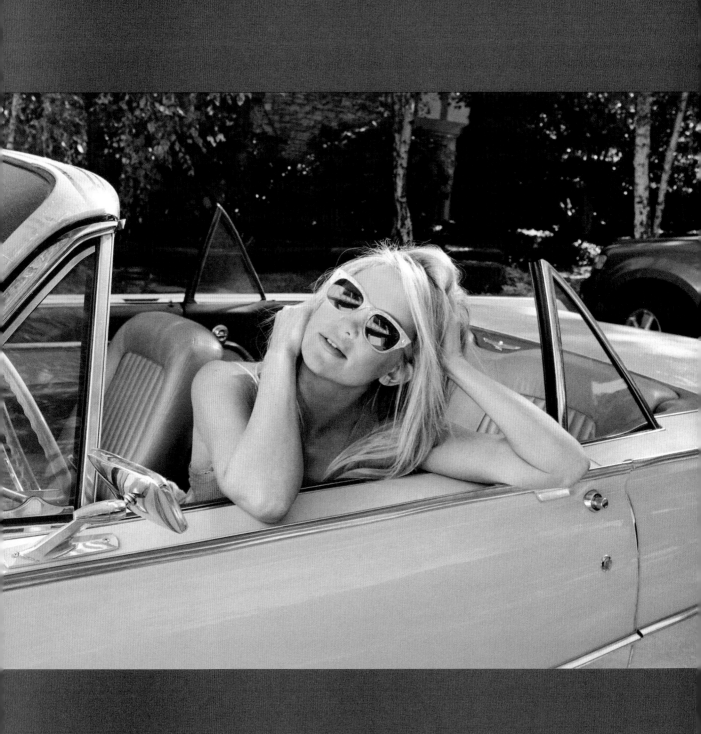

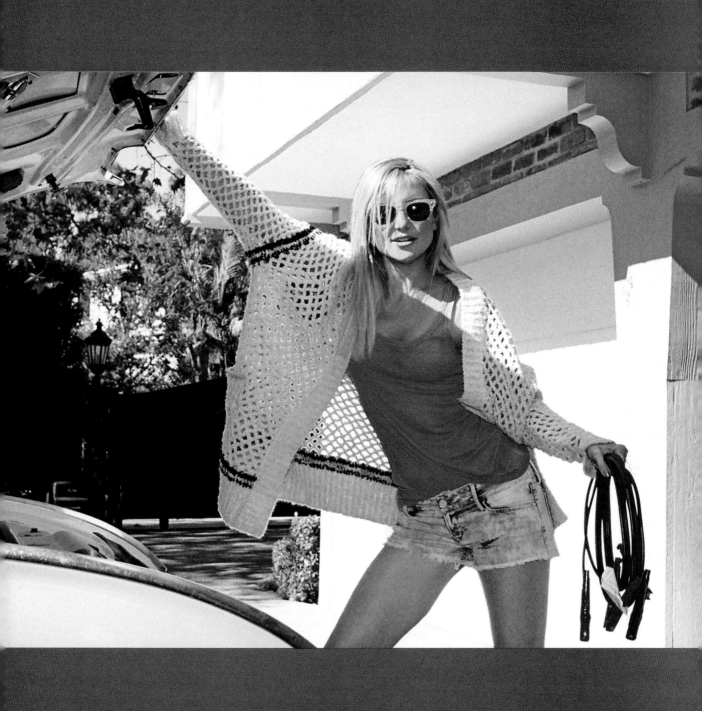

> ## HAVE SOME FUN!
>
> ✳ Visit a butterfly garden ✳ Go fishing ✳ Go sledding
>
> ✳ Laugh at a book of cartoons ✳ Fly a kite ✳ Make an igloo
>
> ✳ Go on a road trip ✳ Finger paint ✳ Build a sand castle
>
> ✳ Pick apples, strawberries, or flowers ✳ Carve a pumpkin
>
> ✳ Remember to smile

Scientists tell us we are driven to seek pleasure—that's the dopamine and endorphins that feel so good. But if we are not present enough to connect to pleasure, we will be like lab rats, continuing to hit the sugar button without ever experiencing the sweet sensation itself. Or the sex addict who gets stuck in the cycle of always hunting down sex instead of enjoying the ride for its own sake.

In order for us to really have pleasure, to truly sink into it in a satisfying way, we need to be spontaneous, relaxed, and open to it. What comes to mind? Play! Fun! Remember being a kid and how satisfying it was to play with your friends? How freeing it was to run around, paint with your hands, and wiggle down a slide? How you didn't have to even think about playing—it was completely natural! Well it's obviously harder to maintain a sense of spontaneous playfulness as we get older, but it's not impossible.

Finding pleasure is enjoying the process and not being attached to the outcome. When we are attached to the outcome, we often set ourselves up for disappointment. This doesn't mean you can't have a lot of what you want—but the picket fence may not happen.

Being spontaneous and open is less about letting go of control than it is about stopping the judgment. We often have an inner voice telling us how to behave: *Don't be silly, That's stupid, How embarrassing,* and so on and so forth. Can't you hear that voice? We've all heard it, but why do we give it any power?

I remember when I went from elementary school to middle school. On the elementary school playground, it was all reckless abandon, boys and girls running around like wild jungle creatures. Then suddenly, as if overnight, we arrived at middle school, and suddenly the girls were hush-hushing in small groups, accusingly staring at other small groups. (The boys were still running around like wild animals.) All at once, the judgments seem to have moved in and clamped down on all our fun. On the one hand, this is a natural part of maturing. But what a loss! And is it really necessary? Don't you think we can do without the judgment and go more with the silly? As my mom would say, if it rains, go take off your shoes and stick your feet in the mud!

I'm all for silliness. It clears the head and lifts the heart!

And at the other end of the fun spectrum is sex. Yes, I said it out loud. Sex is a natural, instinctive, and wholly necessary sensual pleasure. And it's often something we deny ourselves because of a long list of excuses—starting with *I'm tired* and *I'm not in the mood* and ending with *I don't have a partner*. Well let's loosen up, ladies.

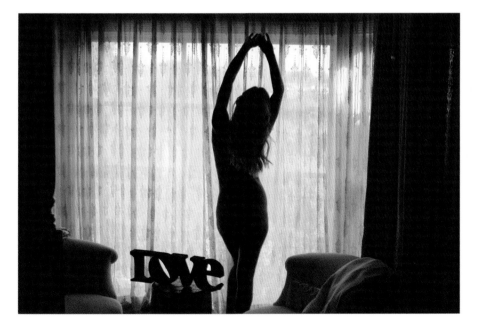

Now might be a good time to talk about my pole dancing: I just started doing it again and I can't believe how much fun it is! Before you jump to any conclusions, let me first say pole dancing is not about showing it off. It's also not about dancing for anyone. It's about connecting with your sensual self—moving in ways that open you up and your own sensual/sexual energy and honoring it for yourself. You rediscover things about your body that you never knew, which is so freeing. It's also a built-in physical challenge. You don't feel the workout while you are dancing—you feel it afterward in your core, arms, and butt. It feels so good to move with music and feel absolute feminine energy. When I practice with other women in a class situation, it's a huge wake-up call to how all women have the power to be sensual and sexy. We all have different bodies, shapes, and ways of being sensual. Sometimes the most sensual woman in the room is the least likely person! If a woman is connected to her own individual beauty, she looks and moves in her own powerful way. How enthralling!

So seek out your own pleasures, let yourself get silly, and play!

Be Content

AN ESSENTIAL INGREDIENT of happiness is being aware enough of what we have in our lives so that we are not on an endless mental quest for what we wish we had. We are all motivated by luxury today—it is all around us and constantly on offer in so may ways. Beautiful things are nice because, well, they are beautiful. But it is important to remind ourselves that we have so much to be grateful for in our lives already, even without the latest luxury goods.

This may sound counterintuitive, but there is happiness in simplicity. By simplifying our lives, boiling our possessions down to what we really need and what really matters to us, there is level of contentment that can be found.

And there is a purity in this contentment too—so that when you look around and see the things in your home, in your life, you know they are there because they have meaning or they are useful.

Maybe with your emerging mindfulness practice, you've already begun to think more about what you are grateful for. There's something about staying present that allows us to treasure what's right in front of us instead of triggering those thoughts of the future or regrets in the past. Meditation also encourages us to be more aware of our attachment to things—how important are all of our material possessions? At the end of the day, aren't our lives more meaningful than the things we surround ourselves with?

Here are some reminders for connecting with this spirit of contentment/gratefulness.

1. Stop judging or criticizing yourself.

2. Stop comparing yourself to others.

3. If you feel bad, don't try to fill the discomfort by buying something.

4. Resist "When I . . . then I" thinking.

5. Be grateful for what you do have.

6. Look for the silver lining in difficult situations.

Being content will naturally emerge from your mindfulness practice, but keeping these six tips in mind will remind you of all that you have to be thankful for in your life.

DRAWING BOARD:
GRATEFULNESS

Make a list of all that comes to mind when you think, *I am grateful for*. . .

_____

_____

_____

_____

_____

_____

_____

_____

_____

_____

_____

_____

_____

_____

_____

_____

_____

_____

_____

_____

_____

What Matters Most

FOR MANY PEOPLE, myself included, a bigger, richer level of happiness comes when we connect with a larger purpose in our lives.

For me, that's my family. I think of them when I wake up in the morning and when I go to bed at night. Like I said, I am a driven person, and my career matters to me. But nothing matters more than being able to share my time and energy with those I love.

Understanding what matters most means asking yourself questions that reveal what is meaningful to you. Take a look at the list below and think about your answers. Then rank the items from 1 to 10, 1 being the most important and 10 being the least important. Be honest with yourself.

THE "WHAT MATTERS TO ME" LIST

* Being in a committed relationship with my partner/spouse
* Raising my children
* Helping or protecting others
* Supporting change in the world
* Achieving success in my career
* Making a lot of money
* Giving back to society
* Creating art to inspire or motivate others
* Solving social problems
* Having fun

This list is not meant to be ranked according to any philosophical value. All of the items have meaning, contribute meaning, and make meaning. It's up to you to define what matters most to you. You can't focus on all of them all of the time. So maybe for now, just ask yourself, what do you want to focus on? How do you want to ground yourself? What are you comfortable with waiting for?

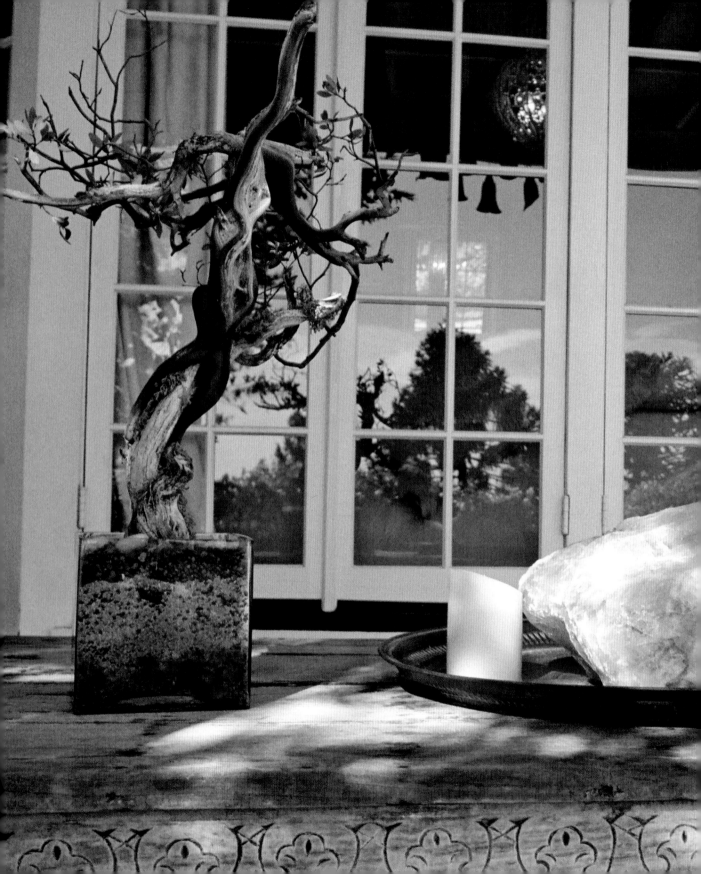

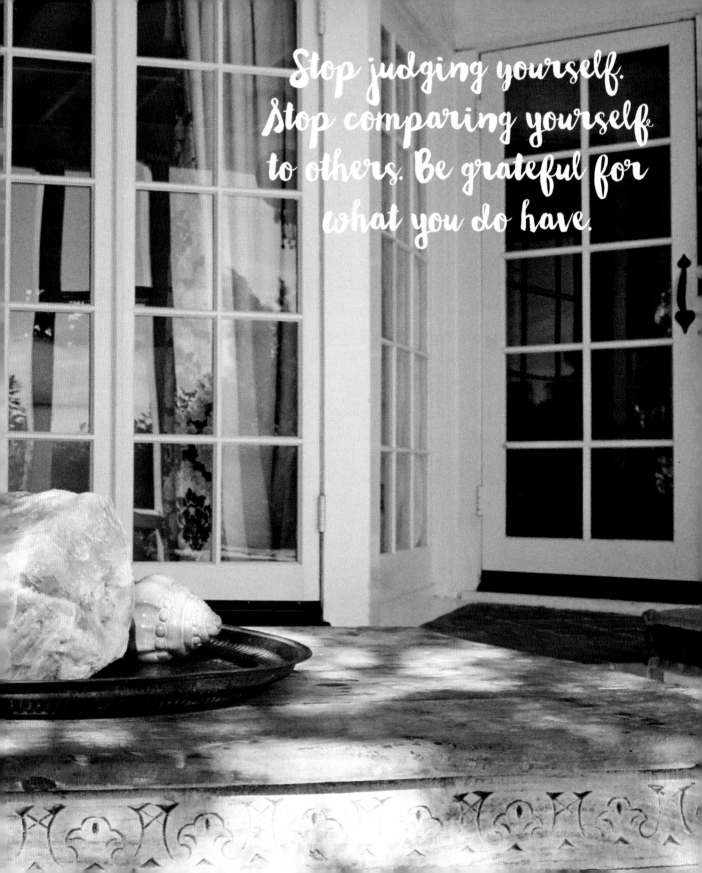

Stop judging yourself.
Stop comparing yourself
to others. Be grateful for
what you do have.

———

Your Drawing Board: Simplify

CONTENTMENT COMES FROM simplifying your life. When I want to clean up my life, I clear out the clutter. I go through my closets and those of my kids. I look throughout my house for "stuff" I no longer want or need. Then I call Goodwill or another charity organization that funnels that stuff to the homeless or other people in need. I also set aside days when I don't go out at all, and stay off the Internet. This time away from social interaction helps me pause and touch down inside of myself. I'm not always the extroverted person people see from the outside. I have a strong introverted side that needs to be nurtured. When I make space and time for that part of myself, it's like coming home.

Here are some suggestions for simplifying your own life.

1. Clean out your closets, basement, or attic.
2. Create a stuff-free zone in your apartment or house where there are no adornments at all.
3. Find space in your day or week when you don't "do" anything. This could be for meditation, rest, or simply staring at a wall or out the window.
4. Carve out quiet time in your home with no interruptions from the Internet, TV, or other media.

When I give myself space—from things, from doing, from wanting—I gain a real sense of freedom. I find that this space is where I become creative and replenish my energy.

Now, take your **Drawing Board** and create a plan for how you will give yourself some "free space" using the guidelines above.

Authenticity

BEING AUTHENTIC TO myself is my own test for whether I am living my own life, making my own decisions, or if, for one reason or another, I am motivated by those other than me. But it's not always easy. In fact, I've made plenty of decisions—about work or relationships—that went against my own values. Sometimes I know right away. Other times it takes me a while. It's not the time lost that matters; it's my understanding and acknowledging my own mistake. Owning your mistakes is a huge part of being authentic.

You live and you learn. You make mistakes, you move on. This is all about becoming an authentic person. No one can tell you how to live or the right way to live. It's all about who you are to yourself. In this way, we are a living testament of the lessons we learn. Yes, being true to ourselves helps us build integrity, that inner strength and solidity that lets us know that no matter what happens, we can count on ourselves. But over time, it's owning our stories that really enables us to live authentically.

Yes, being true to ourselves helps us build integrity, that inner strength and solidity that lets us know that no matter what happens, we can count on ourselves.

BACK TO THE DRAWING BOARD:
COME CLEAN AND MOVE ON

What does being authentic mean to you? Take five minutes and freewrite or just think about your response.

_____

_____

_____

_____

Next, write down five things you've done or decisions you've made that you feel shame or embarrassment about.

_____

_____

_____

What is at the root of the shame? Did someone get hurt by your action or decision? Did you hurt yourself? How?

_____

_____

_____

_____

Finally, accept what you did and know that this behavior or choice does not represent who you are but rather what you did.

Can you forgive yourself for not being perfect?

Sometimes, shifting our viewpoint on ourselves allows us to see that we are not the sum of our mistakes but simply imperfect people doing the best we can.

"LIFE IS A VERB!"

Charlotte Perkins Gilman (1860–1935), author of the great short story "The Yellow Wallpaper" and one of the first American feminist writers, said this in response to a Victorian-era doctor who told her to lie down for two hours before each meal and restrict her intellectual activity to no more than two hours a day. This quote inspires me every day! So next time someone tells you to be quiet, stand still, or stop working, do the opposite:

✳ Use your mind ✳ Laugh a lot ✳ Give to others
✳ Tell the truth ✳ Love always ✳ Pause ✳ Trust yourself
✳ Create fun ✳ Let go ✳ Be yourself

I've arrived at a place in my life where I realize I am *pretty happy*. It's actually not a place at all, but a constant journey and a state of mind.

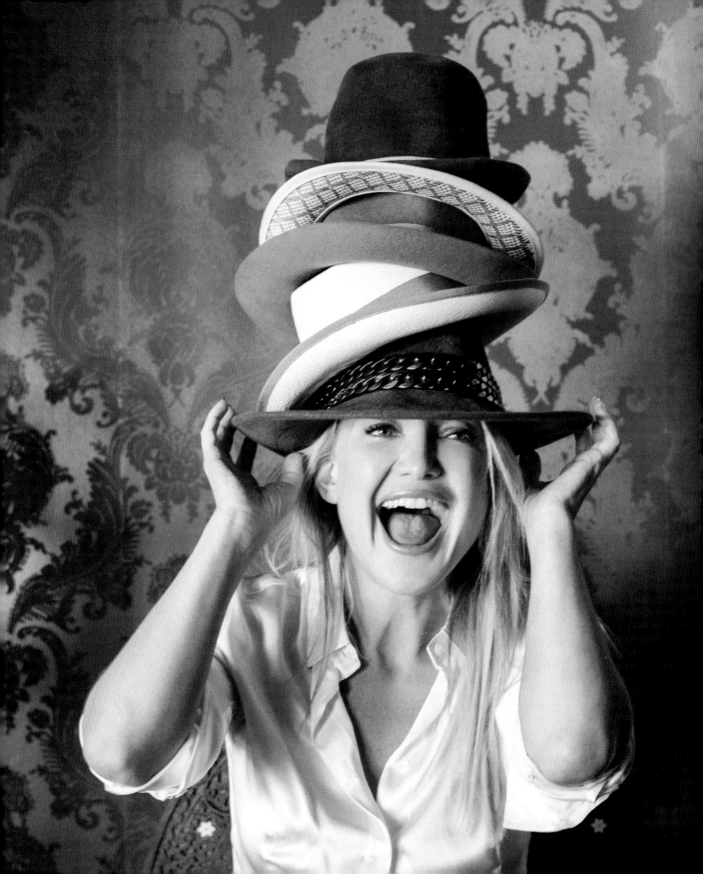

PART THREE

LIVING BODY SMART

We are all body smart. We all have the capacity and the potential to nurture this intuitive relationship with our bodies, calm our minds, and become empowered to steer our lives in the direction of our dreams. To me, that's what living smart is all about. Let's see how to do that on a daily basis.

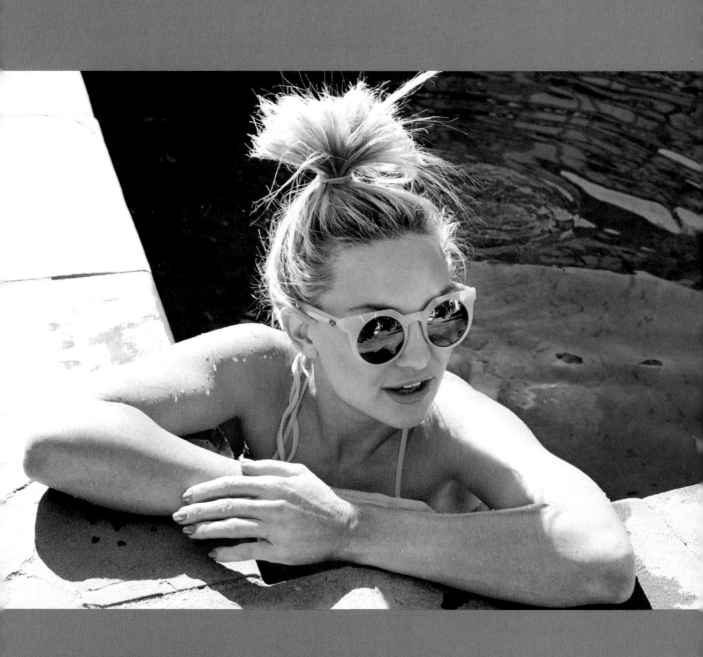

CHAPTER NINE

MAKING IT REAL, MAKING IT WORK

L IVING IN SYNC with your body, finding that intuitive relationship with yourself, and learning to trust your inner voice is all part of the master plan to finding your own pretty happy. I hope that by sharing my own experience and some of my tips and tools for eating clean and getting the exercise I need to feel well will help you on your journey. I hope you can embrace forgiveness and let yourself relax. I also hope you understand that living in a way that builds true inner health begins with nutrition and exercise, includes a regular meditation practice, and always circles back to your Drawing Board.

Take a minute or so to look back at your Drawing Board. What patterns do you see? Where are your highs and lows during the week? Do particular challenges stand out at certain times? It's super important to stay connected to all of the information you put in your Drawing Board—to become aware of your patterns, your triggers, and your triumphs! Like when you lost that first five pounds? Or meditated three days in a row! This chapter will pull together some of the important strategies I use for sticking with it when I get off course, for motivating myself when I need an extra kick in the butt, and recognizing my accomplishments!

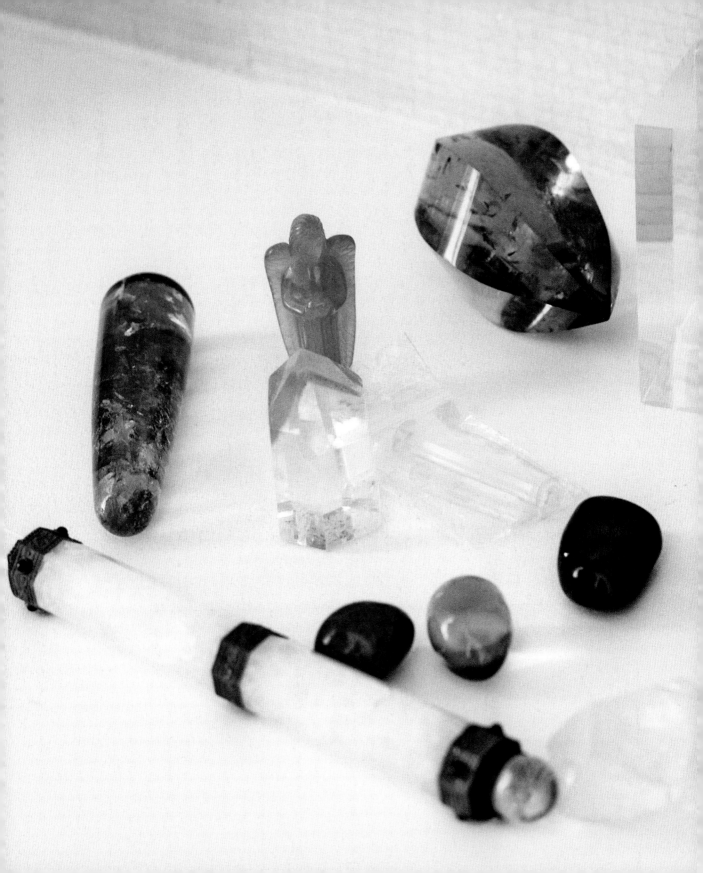

Don't wait for happy to happen.

Motivation Mantra

BEING MOTIVATED TO start something feels easy; staying motivated after the novelty wanes is the hard part. What keeps anyone motivated? I think it comes down to a few important steps:

* **Setting realistic goals.** If your goal is to do your first cleanse, don't set out to do one that is fourteen days long. Try a one- to three-day cleanse to give yourself a realistic chance to experience it successfully. The same is true for weight loss. Good for you that you want to lose a few pounds. Is it more realistic to strive for five pounds in three weeks or ten? When you set your goals at any point in your journey, be realistic.

* **Remind yourself of your goals.** Day in and day out of our busy lives, goals that were once clear can become fuzzy if we don't remind ourselves of them. This is where I become a Post-it fanatic! I literally put sticky notes on my desk computer, on the mirror in my bathroom, on the refrigerator, and in my car. Anywhere I can see them—I also write down my goals and an affirmation to make the reminder even sweeter!

* **Create a circle of love.** Okay. This might sound a little "flower power," but just try it. Think about those people you love, the ones you go to with even the most inane details of your life. In your Drawing Board, create a circle of all those who love you and will root you on. Let them know about the changes you are trying to make in your life. Share with them, ask for their support, and turn to them to help you stay accountable.

* **Acknowledge your progress.** Just as you want to let go of your mistakes, you want to be your own inner cheerleader. Think about all the awesome things you're doing! When you meet a goal, give yourself a big pat on the back! Remind yourself of all that you've accomplished.

* **Don't get hung up on setbacks.** Chill. Forgive yourself. Recognize the mistake or the one, two, or four days of eating like a maniac, and then just get back to your Drawing Board and reset. Make it easy, not an all-or-nothing fight with yourself.

You're in charge of you. Give yourself the opportunity to live the way you want and the room to be imperfect.

We all like our routines. We do them automatically—which means we don't have to think about them. So yes, changing them takes time, energy, and focus. But this time, this way of changing your daily routine is so worth it!

Troubleshooting the Pitfalls

LIFE IS ALWAYS going to get in the way of our best intentions and most well-made plans. That's just a fact. But I've learned a few ways to get back to my Drawing Board more quickly by recognizing certain triggers that tend to set me, and most people, off. Here they are.

* **Low blood sugar.** As soon as our blood sugar drops, our brains take over, driving us to put something into our bodies that will raise the blood sugar in order to get back in metabolic balance. But often the result is reaching for the wrong kind of fix—candy, potato chips, ice cream, a sweet coffee drink. Listen to your body and try to recognize its signals of lowering blood sugar before the situation becomes dire.

* **Stress.** Stress is an inevitable part of our lives, but we can learn to manage it so that it doesn't blindside us. What happens when you are stressed? Do you eat? Withdraw? Get really anxious and can't sleep? Knowing your own signs of mounting stress will help you stay aware of when you need to increase your exercise and/or meditation. Eat more clean or do a cleanse, take more time for you and doing something outside that you really love.

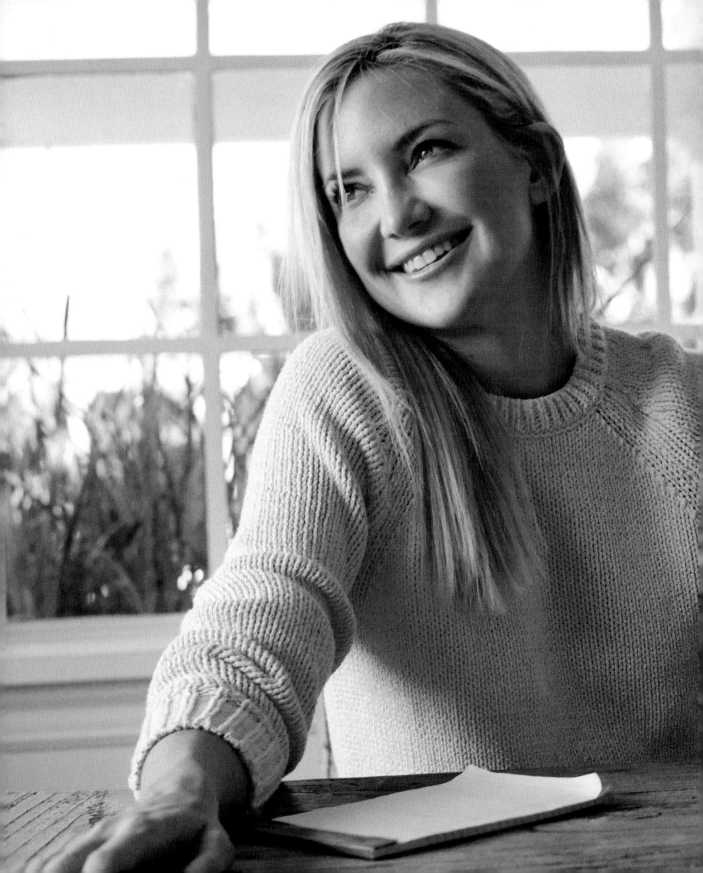

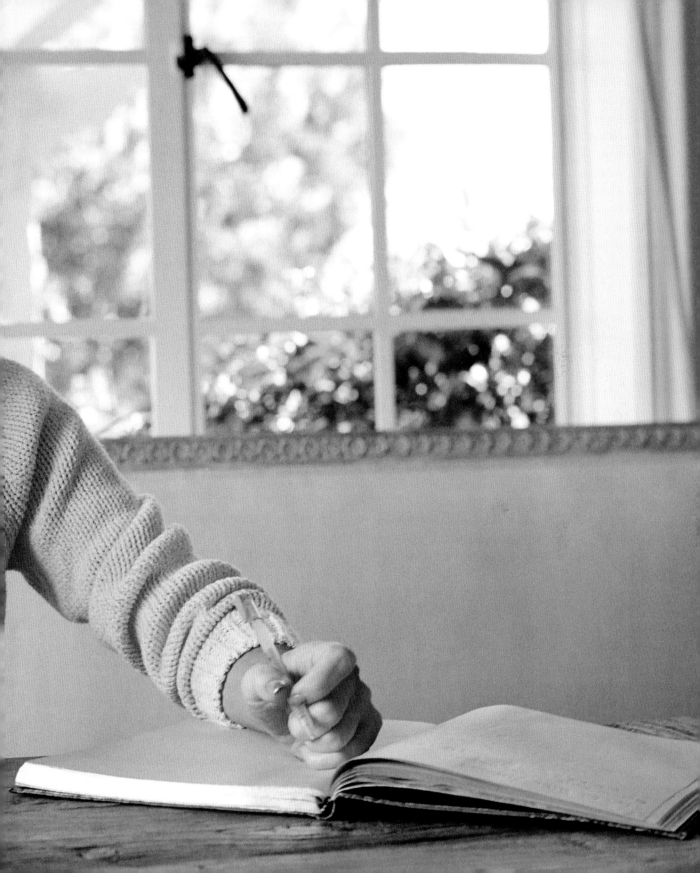

✳ **Hunger.** Don't let yourself get too hungry. This is why I recommend eating three meals and two snacks. If you're hungry, you not only will trigger low blood sugar but end up eating way past being full as well.

✳ **Travel and vacations.** It's hard to eat clean outside of your own safe kitchen when you're on the road, in the air, or on vacation in a hotel. My best advice here is to relax. Try to eat as clean as possible, but don't go crazy in either direction. Don't go to an extreme where you don't enjoy yourself, and don't go hog wild and eat everything in sight! Trust that when you get back home, you can and will reset, with a cleanse or regular clean eating. The same goes for when you are eating at a restaurant or going to a party. Stay away from the extremes and trust your ability to reset.

Prepare and Plan

THESE ARE TWO *P*'s that sound boring, but trust me, they are really important. When you prepare for your week, you set yourself up for success.

1. Shop well.
2. Have your clean foods on hand.
3. Do your bulk prep.

You also will benefit from planning out as many of your meals as possible. If you're doing bulk prep for three meals, you can build off them (see chapter 10 for some sample meal suggestions).

Here's a Grocery List to help you organize your shopping.

GROCERY LIST

Whole Grains
- ◯ Brown rice
- ◯ Brown rice wraps
- ◯ Buckwheat soba noodles
- ◯ Gluten-free flour or pancake mix
- ◯ Popcorn kernels
- ◯ Quinoa
- ◯ Steel-cut oats
- ◯ Whole-grain or gluten-free pasta

Produce
- ◯ Apples
- ◯ Arugula
- ◯ Asparagus
- ◯ Avocado
- ◯ Bananas
- ◯ Beets
- ◯ Bell peppers (red, green, yellow, orange)
- ◯ Berries
- ◯ Bok choy
- ◯ Broccoli
- ◯ Carrots
- ◯ Celery
- ◯ Cucumbers
- ◯ Fennel
- ◯ Kale
- ◯ Kiwi
- ◯ Lemons and limes
- ◯ Mangoes
- ◯ Mixed greens
- ◯ Mushrooms
- ◯ Onions
- ◯ Pears
- ◯ Plums
- ◯ Potatoes
- ◯ Radishes
- ◯ Red cabbage
- ◯ Romaine lettuce
- ◯ Spinach
- ◯ Sweet potatoes
- ◯ Tomatoes
- ◯ Zucchini

Dairy
- ◯ Feta cheese
- ◯ Kefir
- ◯ Soy or almond milk

Proteins
- ◯ Beans (black, kidney, pinto)
- ◯ Chicken breast
- ◯ Chickpeas
- ◯ Edamame
- ◯ Eggs
- ◯ Flank steak
- ◯ Lentils
- ◯ Quinoa
- ◯ Salmon
- ◯ Tempeh
- ◯ Tofu
- ◯ Tuna

Herbs and Spices
- ◯ Basil (fresh)
- ◯ Black pepper
- ◯ Chili powder
- ◯ Cilantro (fresh)
- ◯ Cinnamon
- ◯ Coriander
- ◯ Cumin
- ◯ Ginger (fresh)
- ◯ Garlic (fresh)

Miscellaneous
- ◯ Agave nectar
- ◯ Almond butter
- ◯ Almond milk
- ◯ Avocado oil
- ◯ Balsamic vinegar
- ◯ Coconut oil
- ◯ Dijon mustard
- ◯ Herbal tea
- ◯ Olive oil
- ◯ Raisins
- ◯ Red wine vinegar
- ◯ Sesame seeds
- ◯ Sliced almonds
- ◯ Tahini
- ◯ Tamari
- ◯ Tomato paste, tomato sauce
- ◯ Walnuts

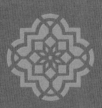

CHAPTER TEN

A WEEK IN
THE LIFE

I WANTED TO SHARE with you a sample week that's typical of my schedule when I'm home in Los Angeles.

Each morning, after I get the kids off to school, I try to do a quick meditation, and sometimes I even get in a meditation class—a luxury for me. You'll see that I build off of my go-to foods, after bulk-prepping on Sundays. I allow some room for grabbing a quick lunch or dinner with friends. Some days I do a strenuous workout; other days I walk or hike with a friend and fit in exercise that way. I would say on average I work out at least four or five days a week—which keeps me in shape and feeling energetic and clearheaded. Right before I go to bed, I try to do another short meditation—this sends me into a peaceful slumber.

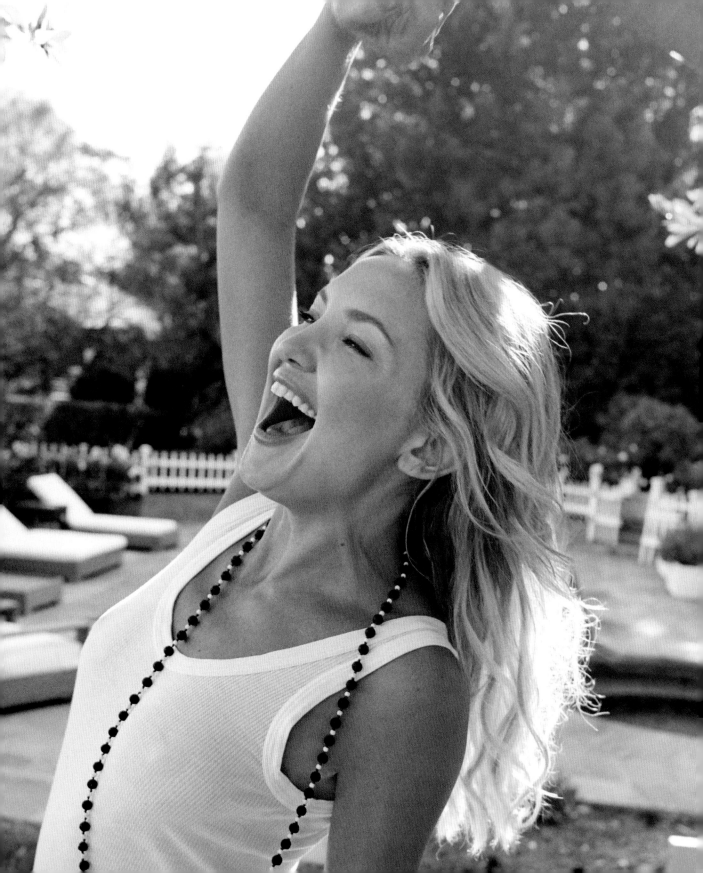

But let me be honest here: this is kind of an ideal week for me. Though I really try to follow this type of schedule and eat all these wonderful clean and nutritious foods, life (work, kids, my own internal changes) can often intervene. If I miss a meal or eat one that is not that clean, I just try to clean up the next few meals to reset. If I go off track for a few days in a row, I might reset with a quick one- or two-day cleanse.

I also don't usually meditate twice a day, every day. I do what I can and believe that once I'm back, my brain and body will kick in and I'll be back where I started. And as I mentioned earlier, although I love to work out five days a week, sometimes it's just three days. I try not to be hard on myself and trust that even if I fit in fifteen minutes of sit-ups, I'll feel better. Again, it's not all-or-nothing.

This "week in the life" is just a snapshot of how I try to eat well, and take care of my mind and body on a day-to-day basis. As I've said, I'm not perfect, and neither is my life. But hopefully you can glean a sense of the flow of my days, the foods that I enjoy, how I build meals from different bases, and how I always, always touch down with myself on a daily basis.

You can start tracking your days using the Daily Planner on pages 232–233. Please feel free to use my weeklong plan to get started, and look for more creative ideas on the Internet. But remember, this is an ideal!

	SUNDAY	**MONDAY**	**TUESDAY**
	Bulk prep day! Go shopping and get all your ingredients. Plan out three to five lunch and dinner meals. Make sure your favorite breakfast foods and snacks are on hand.	**Exercise:** After dropping kids at school, I do 30 minutes of cardio like Spinning.	**Exercise:** Pilates workout for 45 minutes
MORNING MEDITATION		10 minutes in my room	10 minutes in my room
BREAKFAST	Half avocado, half grape-fruit, 2 hard-boiled eggs	Oatmeal with raisins and chopped walnuts	Oatmeal with raisins and chopped walnuts
SNACK	Handful of almonds	Banana	Green power smoothie
LUNCH	Grilled chicken with side of Greek salad (with fresh feta cheese; squeezed lemon as dressing)	Chopped salad with iceberg lettuce, romaine, and other greens; olives; celery; radish; and cucumber (if you want to add protein, add chopped egg white or small portion leftover grilled chicken.)	Leftover lentil tacos and side green salad
SNACK	Hummus and celery sticks	Carrots and celery (with hummus if you feel you need some more protein)	Half avocado
DINNER	Steamed fish in wax paper, broccolini, and sweet peas	Lentil tacos (If I've eaten meat at lunch, I skip it at dinner!)	Butternut squash soup (made with almond milk), sweet potato, side of chopped salad

———

WEDNESDAY	THURSDAY	FRIDAY	SATURDAY
Exercise: With the kids after school, we take the dog for a walk in a nearby canyon.	**Exercise:** pole dancing class	**Exercise:** dance aerobics, such as Tracey Anderson or Body by Simone	**Exercise:** Activites (swimming, basketball, volleyball) with the kids!
11 A.M. meditation class	15 minutes to music	Morning meditation	Morning meditation
Egg burrito	2 soft-boiled eggs, half grapefruit	2 slices whole-grain toast with almond butter	Gluten-free pancakes with the kids!
Banana	Handful of almonds	Watermelon chunks	Homemade trail mix (almonds, cashews, dried unsweetened cranberries)
Grilled salmon over quinoa	Quinoa and avocado salad, topped with some tuna; olive oil and lemon dressing	Leftover stir-fry stuffed into a whole wheat pita	Green smoothie (I'm going out tonight, so I keep it light during the day!)
Handful of almonds or a rice cake with almond butter on top	Banana, hot tea	Celery sticks with hummus	Half avocado with a side of quinoa (to hold me until dinner)
Gluten-free pasta with veggies (zucchini, yellow squash, onions, peppers)	Stir-fry: veggies galore on top of brown rice	Gluten-free pizza night with the kids!	Dinner out with friends!

———

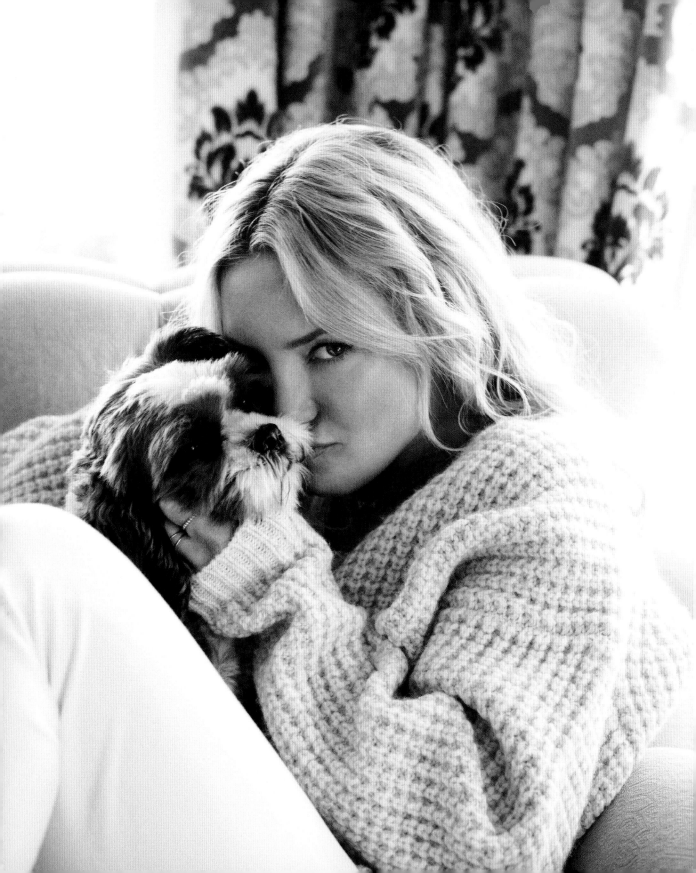

SOME FINAL THOUGHTS

CONGRATULATIONS! YOU'VE ARRIVED! Not at the end of the book, but at the beginning of your own journey. I truly hope that your Drawing Board has become as helpful and empowering as my own is for me. I use it almost every day to dig in and be real with myself. I don't get tired of it because it's like a lifeline to my best self—even when I'm not feeling great. Just knowing that I can dump all my thoughts, feelings, fears, and mistakes into one place gives me a sense of relief and release. It's become the way that I can transform bad to good, jittery to calm, busy to quiet. It's how I retrieve my confidence and resuscitate my energy.

So try it—I hope that you can get to a place where no challenge or problem seems insurmountable, no joy impossible. So relax, enjoy, eat well, and get moving—and I hope you will feel *pretty happy* in no time!

SOME OF MY
FAVORITE BOOKS

As I wrote this book, I consulted many thoughtful, comprehensive books on specific subjects and I'd like to share some of them here. If you're interested in a "deeper dive," these books are a good place to start.

ABOUT FOOD AND NUTRITION

Clean by Alejandro Junger, MD (HarperOne, 2012)

The Everyday Ayurveda Cookbook: A Seasonal Guide to Eating and Living Well by Kate O'Donnell (Shambala, 2015)

The Chopra Center Cookbook: Nourishing Body & Soul by Deepak Chopra, MD (Houghton Mifflin, 2003)

ABOUT MEDITATION AND MINDFULNESS

10 Mindful Minutes: Giving Our Children—and Ourselves—the Social and Emotional Skills to Reduce Stress and Anxiety for Healthier, Happy Lives by Goldie Hawn (Perigee, 2012)

The Book of Awakening: Having the Life You Want by Being Present to the Life You Have by Mark Nepo (Conari, 2000)

The Untethered Soul: The Journey Beyond Yourself by Michael A. Singer (New Harbinger, 2007)

ABOUT FITNESS

The Pilates Body: The Ultimate At Home Guide to Strengthening, Lengthening, and Toning Your Body—Without Machines by Brooke Siler (Harmony, 2000)

Outdoor Fitness: Step Out of the Gym Into the Best Shape of Your Life by Tina Vindum (Falcon Guides, 2009)

ABOUT AYURVEDA

The Wheel of Healing with Ayurveda: An Easy Guide to a Healthy Lifestyle by Michelle Fondin (New World Library, 2015)

ALKALINE AND ACIDIC FOODS LIST

ALKALINE FOODS

Alkalizing Vegetables

Alfalfa

Beet greens

Beets

Broccoli

Cabbage

Carrot

Cauliflower

Celery

Chlorella

Collard greens

Cucumber

Dandelions

Eggplant

Garlic

Green beans

Green peas

Kale

Kohlrabi

Lettuce

Mushrooms

Mustard greens

Onions

Parsnips

Peas

Peppers

Pumpkin

Radishes

Rutabaga

Spinach, green

Spirulina

Sprouts

Sweet potatoes

Swiss chard

Tomatoes

Watercress

Wheatgrass

Alkalizing Asian Vegetables

Daikon

Dandelion root

Kombu

Maitake

Nori

Reishi

Shiitake

Umeboshi

Wakame

Alkalizing Fruits

Apple

Apricot

Avocado

Banana

Berries

Blackberries

Cantaloupe

Cherries, sour

Coconut, fresh

Currants

Dates, dried

Figs, dried

Grapefruit*

Grapes

Honeydew melon

Lemon*

Lime*

Muskmelon

Nectarine*

Orange*

Although it might seem that fruits containing citric acid would have an acidifying effect on the body, the citric acid actually has an alkalinizing effect in the system.

Peach

Pear

Pineapple

Raisins

Raspberries

Rhubarb

Strawberries

Tangerine*

Tomato

Tropical fruits

Watermelon

Alkalizing Protein

Almonds

Chestnuts

Millet

Tempeh (fermented)

Tofu (fermented)

Whey protein powder

Alkalizing Spices and Seasonings

All herbs

Chile pepper

Cinnamon

Curry

Ginger

Miso

Mustard

Sea salt

Tamari

Miscellaneous Alkalizing Foods

Alkaline antioxidant water

Apple cider vinegar

Bee pollen

Fresh fruit juice

Green juices

Lecithin granules

Mineral water

Molasses, blackstrap

Probiotic cultures

Soured dairy products

Stevia

Veggie juices

ACIDIC FOODS

Acidifying Vegetables

Corn

Lentils

Olives

Winter squash

Acidifying Fruits

Blueberries

Canned or glazed fruits

Cranberries

Currants

Plums*

Prunes*

Acidifying Grains and Grain Products

Amaranth

Barley

Bran, oat

Bran, wheat

Bread

Corn

Cornstarch

Crackers, soda

Flour, wheat

Flour, white

Hemp seed flour

Kamut

Macaroni

Noodles

Oatmeal

Oats (rolled)

Quinoa

Rice (all)

Rice cakes

Rye

Spaghetti

Spelt

Wheat

Wheat germ

Although it might seem that fruits containing citric acid would have an acidifying effect on the body, the citric acid actually has an alkalinizing effect in the system.

Acidifying Beans and Legumes

Almond milk

Black beans

Chickpeas

Green peas

Kidney beans

Lentils

Pinto beans

Red beans

Rice milk

Soy milk

Soybeans

White beans

Acidifying Dairy

Butter

Cheese

Cheese, processed

Ice cream

Ice milk

Acidifying Nuts and Butters

Cashews

Legumes

Peanuts

Peanut butter

Pecans

Tahini

Walnuts

Acidifying Animal Protein

Bacon

Beef

Carp

Clams

Cod

Corned beef

Fish

Haddock

Lamb

Lobster

Mussels

Oyster

Pork

Salmon

Sardines

Sausage

Scallops

Shrimp

Tuna

Turkey

Veal

Venison

Acidifying Fats and Oils

Avocado oil

Butter

Canola oil

Corn oil

Hemp seed oil

Flax oil

Lard

Olive oil

Safflower oil

Sesame oil

Sunflower oil

Acidifying Sweeteners

Carob

Corn syrup

Sugar

Acidifying Alcohol

Beer

Hard liquor

Spirits

Wine

Miscellaneous Acidifying Foods

Cocoa

Coffee

Ketchup

Mustard

Pepper

Soft drinks

Vinegar

DAILY PLANNER

MY DAY

TIME	EXERCISE	ME TIME	MEDITATION
7:00 A.M.			
8:00 A.M.			
9:00 A.M.			
10:00 A.M.			
11:00 A.M.			
12:00 P.M.			
1:00 P.M.			
2:00 P.M.			
3:00 P.M.			
4:00 P.M.			
5:00 P.M.			
6:00 P.M.			
7:00 P.M.			

DATE   /   /

BREAKFAST	SNACK	LUNCH	DINNER

ACKNOWLEDGMENTS

No one writes a book alone, and this one is no exception. I wish to thank the many people, voices, experts, and inspiring sources who have helped me shape my ideas for this book.

I would like to thank Carrie Thornton, my editor extraordinaire, whose passion and vision motivated me to write this book.

Thank you to Cait Hoyt at CAA, my stellar agent; Madeleine Ali, my second hand, brain, and heart; Billie Fitzpatrick, my writing partner; and Darren Ankenman, aka Uncle Darren, who has been documenting my life (and my kids' lives) for over fifteen years.

Thank you to Sophie Lopez, my partner in crime—in fashion and life. To Eli Levy, PhD—my gratitude for him is immeasurable; he is the reason I have the confidence to even share my ideas.

Thanks, too, to Nicole Stuart.

I would also like to thank the entire Dey Street Books team, including Sean Newcott, Lynn Grady, Michael Barrs, Shelby Meizlik, Heidi Richter, Jeanne Reina, Mumtaz Mustafa, Nyamekye Waliyaya, Ivy McFadden, Lucy Albanese, Suet Chong, Sun Young Park, and Paul Kepple.

And most important, my Mom and Pa, for their continuous love, support, and encouragement.

ABOUT THE AUTHOR

KATE HUDSON is a Golden Globe Award winner and Academy Award–nominated actress, producer, and entrepreneur. She is best known for her roles in *Almost Famous*, *How to Lose a Guy in 10 Days*, and *Bride Wars*, which she also produced. On television, Kate received critical acclaim for her guest-star appearance on the hit show *Glee*. She is the voice of Mei Mei in *Kung Fu Panda 3*.

Kate's love of design and fashion has seen her become an international style icon and muse for some of the world's top designers. She has also been featured in many global advertising campaigns, most recently the renowned Campari Calendar, and has been the face of major retail brands, including Ann Taylor and Almay.

In 2013, Kate cofounded Fabletics (fabletics.com), a line of stylish and affordable activewear designed to inspire and empower women to get physically fit and as a way of living that promotes health, community, and passion.

Kate lives in Los Angeles with her two sons.

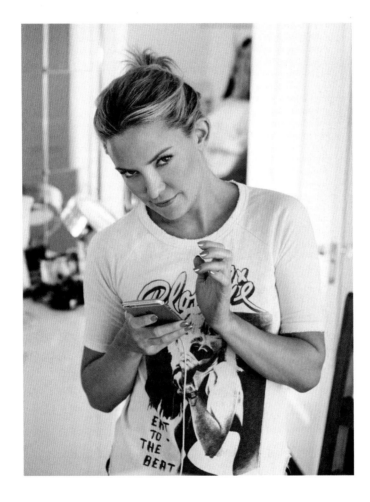